Fit Cuisine

Healthy Food Made Simple

Francesca Pucher

iUniverse, Inc.
Bloomington

Fit Cuisine
Healthy Food Made Simple

iUniverse books may be ordered through booksellers or by contacting:

iUniverse
1663 Liberty Drive
Bloomington, IN 47403
www.iuniverse.com
1-800-Authors (1-800-288-4677)

ISBN: 978-1-4759-0710-0 (sc)
ISBN: 978-1-4759-0711-7 (ebk)

Printed in the United States of America

iUniverse rev. date: 04/30/2012

Contents

Dedication vii

Quick and Healthy Breakfast Meals

Berry Smoothie 3
Layered Fruit Salad 4
Boston Marathon Breakfast 5
Quinoa Breakfast 6

Healthy Soups and Hearty Stews

Tuscan Tortellini Soup with Chicken Sausage 9
Italian Lentil Soup 11
Eggplant and Ravioli Soup 12
Asparagus Soup 13
Sweet Potato Soup 14
Butternut Squash and Apple Soup 15
Non-Cream-of-Vegetable Soup 16
Baked Chicken and Vegetable Stew 17
Italian Wedding Soup 18
Sausage and Pepper Stew with Brown Rice 19
Barley Soup with Carrots and Chickpeas 20
Low-Fat Turkey Chili 21

Healthy Salads and Vegetable Dishes

Presentation Salad 25
White and Green Bean Salad 26
Whole Wheat Pasta Salad 27
Arugula Salad with Slivered Almonds, Diced Apples, Goat
    Cheese, and Balsamic 28

Holiday Sweet Potato Salad 29
Grilled Steak and Vegetable Salad 30
Chicken Salad 31
Papaya—Avocado Salad.. 32
Cucumber Roasted Pepper and Tomato Salad........................ 33
Spinach and Goat Cheese Salad... 34
Pesto Shrimp and Rice Salad 35
Chicken, Tomato, and Broccoli Salad.................................... 36
Asparagus with Roasted Almonds.. 37
Whipped Cauliflower.. 38
Whipped Sweet Potatoes 39
Roasted Eggplant Spread... 40
Sweet Carrots 41
Sautéed Green Beans with Cherry Tomatoes 42

Healthy and Simple Pastas

Baked Whole Wheat Rotini with Squash............................... 45
Cavatelli with Sautéed Spinach, White Beans, and Cherry Tomatoes... 46
Elbow Pasta Baked with Vegetables....................................... 47
Spinach, Tomato, and Whole Wheat Pasta 48
Lasagna Rolls.. 50
Lemon-Infused Linguine... 51
Escarole with White Beans 52
Roasted Vegetables with Whole Wheat Pasta 54
Sautéed Zucchini, Eggplant, and White Beans with Whole
    Wheat Pasta 55
Shrimp and Linguini with Spinach.. 56
Spaghetti Pie 57
Low-Fat Spinach Lasagna 59
Stuffed Shells with Zucchini Topping.................................... 60
Whole Wheat Baked Ziti... 62
Whole Wheat Orecchiette Pasta with Garlic Oil and Pine Nuts 64

Vegetarian and Fish Dishes

Baked Eggplant Parmesan 67
Grilled Vegetable Bake.. 68

Baked Zucchini Parmesan 69
Black Bean Burgers 70
Easy-Baked Salmon with Fresh Mango Salsa 72
Lemon Pepper Panko Salmon 73
Pesto-Topped Grilled Squash.. 74
Quinoa and Black Beans 75
Ratatouille... 76
Vegetable and Rice Sauté.. 77
Whole Grain Pizza Crust.. 78
Zucchini, Squash, and Tomato Bake...................................... 79

Something-Other-Than-Chicken Dishes

Turkey Spinach Meatballs... 82
Spinach and Goat Cheese Turkey Burgers............................... 84
Italian Turkey Meat Loaf.. 86
Small Thanksgiving Dinner: 88
Stuffed Zucchini Boats.. 89
Stuffed Acorn Squash... 90
Stuffed Peppers with Quinoa 91
Pork Stir-Fry with Noodles... 92
Marinated Italian Pork Loin 93
Low-Fat Turkey Bolognese... 94
Crusted Pork Loin with Tomato 95
Chicken Sausage Ragout 96
Brown Rice Bake with Meatballs 97
Healthy Sausage and Peppers with Brown Rice....................... 98

Endless Chicken Dishes

Quinoa with Spinach, Chicken, and Feta Cheese 101
Rotisserie Chicken and Fresh Vegetable Bake......................... 102
Spaghetti Squash with Chicken, Zucchini, Sun-Dried Tomatoes,
    and String Beans 103
Pesto Baked Chicken with Roasted Peppers............................ 105
Baked Chicken Parmesan 106
Broccoli, Chicken, and Rice Bake.. 107

Balsamic Chicken with Mushrooms, Tomatoes, Olives, Basil, and Goat Cheese 108
Grilled Chicken Greek Salad 109
Chicken Breasts Stack with Mozzarella and Tomato 110
Chicken Roll-Up with Goat Cheese and Asparagus 111
Chicken with Mango and Peach Salsa 112
Stuffed Chicken with Spinach, Roasted Red Peppers, and Mozzarella 113
Broccoli and Chicken Pie 114
Chicken Breasts with Roasted Red Peppers, Artichokes, and Sun-Dried Tomatoes 116

Healthy and Simple Almost-Desserts

Piña Colada Cake 119
Coconut Cookies 122
Applesauce 123
Baked Apple Crisp 124
Dark Chocolate Chip Cookies 125
Bunny Cupcakes 126
Fresh Fruit with Yogurt Dressing and Angel Food Cake 129
Fit Cuisine Grocery Items 131

Dedication

This book is being dedicated to my mother, without her love, support, and guidance in the kitchen this book would not be what it is today.

1

QUICK AND HEALTHY BREAKFAST MEALS

Berry Smoothie

WHAT YOU WILL NEED:

1 cup low-sugar cranberry juice
1 cup blueberry Greek yogurt
1 small or 1/2 large frozen banana cut into pieces (easiest to cut pieces prior to freezing)
1/2 cup frozen blueberries
4-5 frozen strawberries
2-3 ice cubes

Place each ingredient into a blender and blend until smooth. Pour into frosted glass with a straw and serve.

FIT CUISINE NOTES: 🗒

I love berry smoothies. Use this for breakfast, lunch, or a pre/ post-workout snacks. I love berries, and the Greek yogurt adds just enough thickness to this drink. If you are not a fan of cranberry, you may use raspberry or boysenberry juice instead.

Time: 5 minutes
Serving: 4 3/4 cups

Layered Fruit Salad

WHAT YOU WILL NEED:

1/2-3/4 cup each of strawberries, sliced bananas, blackberries, and blueberries
1/2 cup fat-free or low-fat Greek yogurt
1 tbsp cinnamon
1 tbsp honey
1/2 cup of high-fiber, low-sugar cereal
1/4 cup unsweetened shredded coconut
1/4 cup chopped walnuts or sliced almonds

Mix fruit together and put half of the mixture into a large bowl. Blend yogurt with cinnamon and honey. Spoon half of the yogurt mixture on top of the fruit. Then top with half the cereal, coconut, and walnuts. Repeat the layers with the remaining fruit, yogurt, cereal, coconut, and nuts.

FIT CUISINE NOTES:

This dish is great as breakfast, lunch, or dessert. I actually had this recipe featured on sheknows.com, under healthy breakfast alternatives. This is my go-to meal when I am at work or pressed for time. The kids would like this as well, and they won't even realize how good it is for them.

Time: 5 minutes
Serving: 2

Boston Marathon Breakfast

WHAT YOU WILL NEED:

1/2 cup instant oatmeal made with water
1 tsp natural peanut butter
1 small banana (sliced)

In a microwave-safe bowl place your oatmeal, water, and sliced banana. Heat in the microwave according to package directions. Once complete, take your peanut butter and stir everything together. Eat and enjoy!

FIT CUISINE NOTES:

This was my breakfast of champions throughout my marathon training. I must say, it also became my favorite meal of the day. I love peanut butter and, when you combine it with a banana, *wow,* what a yummy dish! This recipe was given to me by my brother-in-law who is also a fitness trainer. When I saw how it looked, I was not sure—but once I tried it, I was hooked. It became the morning meal that got me across the finish line of the Miami Marathon in 3:39—my official Boston Marathon qualifier. I love this meal because it has everything: complex carbohydrates, good fat, and potassium. I recommend it to a lot of my clients who need a wholesome, healthy, and quick breakfast in the morning.

Time: 2 minutes
Serving: 1

Quinoa Breakfast

WHAT YOU WILL NEED:

1/2 cup cooked quinoa (in water)
2 oz unsweetened Almond Breeze
Dash of cinnamon
1/3 cup fresh berries

Make your quinoa according to the package, and place it in the fridge overnight (for use in the morning). Take your quinoa and place it into a microwave-safe bowl and add your almond breeze and cinnamon. Place in the microwave for about 1 1/2 minutes. Take out, stir, and add your berries. Eat and enjoy.

FIT CUISINE NOTES:

This is a great meal if you want something warm but can't eat gluten, like me. I decided to try this dish because I just love quinoa. You can make a batch and leave it in the refrigerator for a few days—it's always ready to go. What I did with this dish was substitute what I used to use (oatmeal) for a better grain that has more protein and helps me maintain my energy level throughout a long morning of training. Plus, you get calcium from the Almond Breeze, which is dairy-free, and you get antioxidants from all the great berries. I would definitely try this great dish—if you don't want it for breakfast; it makes an awesome snack as well.

Time: 25 minutes (to cook quinoa). If already cooked, 10 minutes in the microwave.
Serving: 1-2

2

HEALTHY SOUPS AND HEARTY STEWS

Tuscan Tortellini Soup with Chicken Sausage

WHAT YOU WILL NEED:

1 package Nature's Promise Italian seasoned sausage (removed from casing and chopped)
1 large can plum tomato (in juice)
1 zucchini, diced
1/2 eggplant, diced
1 squash, diced
1 cup fresh, chopped spinach
1 tsp Mrs. Dash (Italian Medley Blend, no salt)
1 cup fresh tortellini
2 cups organic, low-sodium chicken broth
1 tbsp garlic
2 tbsp olive oil

In a soup pot, sauté olive oil, garlic, and sausage together. Once your sausage starts to cook (which will happen quickly because it's chicken), add your can of plum tomatoes, breaking them apart. Let the whole pot come to a boil and cook for about 15-20 minutes. Add your sliced vegetables and chicken broth along with your seasoning. Let the entire pot come to a boil again for about 10 minutes, then lower the heat to a simmer for another 5. Make sure that your vegetables are cooked before you add the pasta. Let the pasta cook with the soup for about 5 minutes. Lower the heat and serve.

Fit Cuisine Notes:

This is a great and hearty soup. It is also one of my many easy, healthy, one-pot, complete meals that can be lunch or dinner. I really became a fan of chicken sausage and thought it was a nice complement to this soup—it was low in salt and high in flavor. Plus, who doesn't love tortellini? With this dish, you only need a cup, so everyone gets a taste without all the extra calories, plus a sprinkle of Parmesan cheese is a great compliment to this dish as well.

Time: 30-40 minutes
Serving: 4-6

Italian Lentil Soup

WHAT YOU WILL NEED:

1 bag lentils
8 cups water
1 package Italian chicken sausage
1 cup carrots, diced
1 cup celery, diced
1 tbsp garlic, minced
2 tbsp olive oil
1 (15 oz) can diced tomatoes (no salt)
Dash of black pepper
Dash of basil
Dash of red pepper
1 cup green beans, diced

In a large soup pot, sauté your oil, garlic, carrots, and celery. Add in your water, lentils, and green beans; stir together. Let it come to a boil. Once it does, add your sausage (already cooked), canned tomatoes, and seasoning. Reduce the heat to a low simmer for about 25-30 minutes, until the vegetables and lentils are tender. You may need to add a bit more water—if so, add 1 cup at a time. Once it is complete, let it cool and serve.

FIT CUISINE NOTES:

This is a great one-pot meal. It can be made with or without the sausage and, if you want, served on a bed of quinoa or rice. Sprinkle with a bit of parmesan cheese and enjoy.

Time: 1 hour
Serving: 6-8

Eggplant and Ravioli Soup

What You Will Need:

1 (28 oz) can crushed tomatoes with basil
4 cups low-sodium vegetable broth
2 cups water
1 eggplant (zebra peeled and sliced)
1 tbsp olive oil
2 tbsps butter (I Can't Believe It's Not Butter)
2 tbsps garlic, minced
Dash of black pepper
1 package tiny ravioli (found in fresh food section of market)

In a medium-size soup pot, over low heat, cook your oil and butter. While that is setting up, peel and chop your eggplant. Add it to the pot along with your garlic and let it start to get soft. Pour your crushed tomatoes, broth, and water in. Let the entire pot simmer for about 5-10 minutes or until the eggplant is soft. Wait to add the pasta until the entire soup is complete. You don't want to have ravioli that burst and ruin the soup. Turn the soup to low and add the pasta. Simmer for 5 minutes and turn off heat, letting it sit.

Fit Cuisine Notes:

You can add any vegetable you want to this (broccoli, zucchini, squash). I actually added a few slices of zucchini and it was great. This is a complete meal, and it's filled with flavor. I like to call it an eggplant parmesan-style soup without all the gooey cheese. Plus, it goes well with a large salad. This is made in one pot, and I love that it can be eaten for lunch the next day.

Time: 30 minutes
Serving: 4-8

Asparagus Soup

WHAT YOU WILL NEED:

1 tbsp extra virgin olive oil
1 small onion, chopped
1 garlic clove, minced
2 1/2 pounds asparagus ends, trimmed and cut into 1 1/2" lengths (fresh or frozen)
4 cups low-sodium chicken broth
Salt and freshly ground white pepper
4 tsps freshly grated parmesan cheese

Heat oil in a saucepan over medium heat. Add onion, garlic, and asparagus to cook, stirring occasionally until onions soften (5-7 minutes). Do not brown. Add broth, bring to a simmer, and cook until asparagus is just tender (about 10 minutes). Remove from heat and carefully puree with a blender or emulsifier. Return to the pan, gently reheat, and season with salt and pepper to taste. Sprinkle each serving with some freshly grated parmesan.

FIT CUISINE NOTES:

I *love* asparagus, but I don't enjoy it in a thick, rich soup. I used chicken broth (but you could use vegetable broth if you want to make it less creamy). It tastes great, but I will say it is nothing like your traditional asparagus soup—it is light and clean tasting. It pairs well with grilled chicken over salad or by itself for lunch.

Time: 30 minutes
Serving: 4

Sweet Potato Soup

WHAT YOU WILL NEED:

4 large, sweet potatoes
2 containers of low-sodium vegetable broth
3 cloves of garlic, minced

Take your sweet potatoes and either roast them or do what I did and flash steam them. To flash steam, you take the potato, puncture holes in it with a fork, and stick it in the microwave for 4-5 minutes on high heat till soft. Do this with all your spuds. While the potatoes are heating, take your soup pot and heat up your broth and garlic. Carefully remove the inside of your potatoes and place it into the pot. Let it simmer for about 20 minutes. Then, using a masher or emulsifier, puree your soup until it is thick and creamy. Heat for a remaining 5 minutes and serve.

FIT CUISINE NOTES: 🖊

This soup is loaded with vitamins and nutrients for the cold weather. Plus, it is super easy to make. I love sweet potatoes—they are a great alternative to white potatoes, and they have a great natural sweetness to them. What is great about this dish is that, if you have leftover sweet potatoes from a holiday meal, it's a great way to use leftovers. It works really well as a starter before a meal or by itself for lunch.

Time: 30-45 minutes
Serving: 4-8

Butternut Squash and Apple Soup

What You Will Need:

1 batch of already-cut butternut squash (or half of a whole one, diced)
3 honey crisp apples (skin removed and sliced)
1 small onion, chopped
1 container of low-sodium vegetable stock (organic)
Dash of thyme
Dash of black pepper
1 tbsp olive oil
1 small container Fage 0% yogurt

Preheat oven to 400. On a baking sheet place your squash, apples, and onions. Coat everything with the thyme, olive oil, and pepper mixture. Place into the oven for about 30 minutes. In a pot, place your vegetable stock and heat. Once heated through, turn on low and simmer until vegetables are done. Take your vegetables and fruit from the oven and place them in the pot of vegetable stock. Let it come to a boil for about 5 minutes so that everything is soft. Take a blender, food processor, or emulsion blender and whip everything together. Remove from heat for and let cool a bit before adding your yogurt. Once cooled, add the yogurt and some more pepper to taste. Whip or stir one last time, heat again, and serve.

Fit Cuisine Notes:

I loved the way this came out when I first made it. It sounds weird, but it is so clean tasting and healthy that you can eat two bowls and not have all the salt and crazy spices. Plus, you get added fiber from the apples and protein from the yogurt. I used yogurt so that I can get a creamy texture without the fat. This was served for our Thanksgiving meal, and the entire family loved it. Now it's a staple in our fall menu.

Time: 30-45 minutes
Serving: 4-6

Non-Cream-of-Vegetable Soup

WHAT YOU WILL NEED:

1 tbsp olive oil
1/2 cup shallots
4 cups low-sodium vegetable broth
1 cup water
2 (12 oz) bags frozen cauliflower, thawed
1 cup red peppers, chopped
1 package silken tofu
1 tbsp white wine vinegar
Dash of black pepper
Dash of sea salt
Dash of nutmeg

In a soup pot sauté your olive oil and shallots until they are translucent. Place your vegetable broth and water into the pot until it simmers. Add your vegetables and wait until they are tender. Using a blender or mixer of choice, puree your soup—either in groups or all together—until it becomes pureed. Once blended, add your tofu and white wine. Pour back into your pot and add your remaining seasonings. Serve with parmesan cheese and enjoy.

FIT CUISINE NOTES:

Make sure you have a large enough blender for this recipe (if not, use a Cuisinart processor or a Ninja). This is a very clean style soup, so you may feel it needs more salt—try not to add much, there is enough in the vegetable broth. Also, this is a great way to enjoy a creamy style soup without all the fat and calories. It pairs well with a turkey sandwich or a large salad (or you could have it by itself for lunch or dinner).

Time: 40-50 Minutes
Serving: 4-8

Baked Chicken
and Vegetable Stew

WHAT YOU WILL NEED:

1 zucchini, diced
1 package chicken breasts
1 jar of Ellie's Stew (gluten-free, low-sodium)
2 squirts of pesto (from a tube)
1 tsp Mrs. Dash (Tomato Basil Garlic Blend)

Preheat oven to 400. In a baking dish, sprinkle your seasoning on both sides of the chicken, top your chicken with your diced zucchini and your jar of stew. Then squirt a small amount of pesto over the chicken mix. Bake in the oven for about 20 minutes, depending on chicken size. Remove from the oven and serve with a side salad or quinoa.

FIT CUISINE NOTES:

I am a huge fan of one-pot, complete meals, and I also love soup. I like my soups to be more than just broth so I can have it for dinner and not feel hungry later on. I also like to cook some of my meals (and my clients' meals) gluten free. I found Ellie's Stew in the market and thought the ingredients were good—all I needed to do was add some more of my favorite vegetables to the dish to make it really nutritious and dense. I love this recipe; it's not just healthy, but quick as well. You can make this in advance or when you get home from a long day; it's that quick and easy.

Time: 30 minutes
Serving: 4-6

Italian Wedding Soup

WHAT YOU WILL NEED:

Meatballs:
1 lb ground turkey (chicken or beef)
1 egg
1 handful Italian-seasoned bread crumb
Dash of parmesan cheese

Soup:
2 containers reduced-sodium chicken broth
5 cups water
2 heads escarole (or 3 lbs spinach)
Dash of pepper
1 tsp Mrs. Dash (Italian Medley Blend)
1/2 lb small-sized pasta (elbow or pastina)

Preheat oven to 400. In a mixing bowl, combine your ground meat and all the meatball ingredients. Take the mixture and make small meatballs with it—you should get about 20 meatballs. Place on a baking sheet and bake for about 20 minutes. While they are baking, take a large soup pot and add your chicken broth and water. Let that come to a boil and add in your spinach or escarole until it wilts down. Then toss in the seasoning and pasta. Let the pasta cook in the soup. Once your pasta is al dente, add your meatballs. Simmer on low heat for about 12 minutes and serve. Plate with fresh parmesan and enjoy.

FIT CUISINE NOTES:

I am a big fan of this soup, and I loved eating it when I was sick. At first, though (when I left home and moved into my own house), I used to eat the canned version. Then I saw how much sodium was in a serving! Let's just say it was way too much for one meal. So I came up with this recipe by deconstructing the canned version. This way I know that what I am eating is healthy, and I can control the salt. Plus, it is a big hit with the family and a great soup to bring to a sick loved one.

Time: 40-50 minutes
Serving: 6-8

Sausage and Pepper Stew
with Brown Rice

WHAT YOU WILL NEED:

1 package chicken sausage, diced (Italian seasoning, Al Fresco or Nature's
    Promise brand)
1 red pepper, chopped
1 yellow pepper, chopped
1 orange pepper, chopped
1 small shallot, chopped
1 can low-salt, stewed tomatoes
1 can low-salt tomato sauce
Dash of basil
Dash of pepper
1 package brown rice
1 tbsp minced garlic
1 tbsp olive oil

In a sauté pan, heat up your garlic and oil. Add to that your diced peppers
and shallots; Sauté with the oil and garlic. Add your stewed tomatoes and
tomato sauce. Let the entire thing cook until the peppers are soft. Add
your diced sausage (it should already be cooked). Simmer for about 10
minutes on medium-low heat. Cook up your rice and add it to the mix of
sausage and pepper. Serve and enjoy.

FIT CUISINE NOTES:

As an Italian, we always had sausage and peppers at gatherings, and
sometimes for Sunday dinner. This is a great low-calorie way to enjoy a
family favorite. Plus, everything is made in one pot on the stove. I love the
chicken sausage in this dish, it has all the flavor pork would have, and it's
already cooked (and it has less fat than the regular sausage you would use
in this dish). I recommend making this dish for a potluck gathering or an
easy weekday supper that everyone will love.

Time: 40 minutes
Serving: 6-8

Barley Soup with Carrots and Chickpeas

What You Will Need:

1/4 cup barley
1 cup carrots, diced
1 cup carrot juice
3 cups water
3 cups chicken stock (low-sodium)
1 (15.5 oz) can chickpeas (rinsed)

In a large soup pot, bring your water and chicken stock to a low simmer. Add your diced carrots and barley, and let them cook until your carrots are tender. Add your juice and chickpeas. Let it all simmer for another 10-15 minutes. Once done, take a masher or emulsifier and whip until the carrots are just about broken. Serve and enjoy.

Fit Cuisine Notes: ✎

I love barley—it is a great alternative to pasta and rice, it contains little gluten, and due to its high fiber content you feel satisfied longer. It is yet another one-pot, complete meal that can be made for dinner one night or used for lunch the next day.

Time: 30-45 minutes
Serving: 4-8

Low-Fat Turkey Chili

What You Will Need:

1 tbsp olive oil
1 tbsp garlic, minced
2 packs ground turkey
6 peppers (mix of yellow, orange, and red)
2 (15.5 oz) cans red kidney beans, drained
1/2 jar tomato sauce
2 (14.5 oz) cans low-salt, diced tomatoes
Dash of chili powder
Dash of black pepper
Dash of crushed red pepper flakes

Slightly coat the bottom of a pot with olive oil, turn the heat on, and sauté your garlic. Add turkey to the pot once your garlic starts to cook. Let the turkey cook all the way through and start cutting your peppers. When the turkey is done, add the peppers, diced tomatoes, and tomato sauce to the pot. Let it simmer until the peppers are tender, then add the beans and spices. Let the pot simmer on low for about 30 minutes and serve.

Fit Cuisine Notes: ✐

Chili is great, but I find that when I order it at a restaurant the spices are too much for me (and it's loaded with salt and extra oil). I wanted my chili to be hearty, not too saucy, spiced just right, with little oil. I wanted to be able to feel well after eating this dish—not too full—so I added small amounts of sauce and chopped my vegetables small as well. I also used only one bean in this dish to make it less filling. I enjoy this dish as is, but some like it with a little brown rice or quinoa—either would be fine. This dish tastes even better the next day.

Time: 30-40 minutes
Serving: 4-8

3

HEALTHY SALADS AND VEGETABLE DISHES

Presentation Salad

WHAT YOU WILL NEED:

1 small can mandarin oranges (drained)
1 English cucumber, sliced
1 package mixed greens
1 endive, sliced
2 tbsps dried Craisins
1 small fennel bulb, chopped
1 tbsp toasted pine nuts

This is a toss-in-one-bowl dish. Add your mixed greens, endive, and fennel. Then toss in your cucumbers, pine nuts, and Craisins. Mix all that together. Layer the mandarin oranges around the bowl for presentation. Serve with your favorite light vinegar or squeezed lemon.

FIT CUISINE NOTES:

I taught my first cooking class how to prepare this salad. It was inspired by a salad my mother-in-law makes during the holidays or fun family get-togethers. I wanted to show clients that it is easy to make a pretty looking salad fast with fruit and a light vinegarette. It was a big hit, and it really does look pretty in a large salad bowl. You can use this as a main weekend dish as well. Add in some grilled shrimp or salmon and you have a light, complete meal in minutes.

Time: 20 minutes
Serving: 6-8

White and Green Bean Salad

What You Will Need:

1 (15.5 oz) can white cannellini beans
1 tbsp red pepper
1 tbsp fresh parsley
1/4 cup diced tomatoes (fresh)
1 tbsp red onion
1 tsp extra virgin olive oil
1 tbsp balsamic vinegar
1 cup green beans
1 tsp herb and spice blend

Drain the can of beans and rinse well in a strainer. Blanch your green beans by boiling them in water until slightly tender. Then place them in an ice bath or a microwave-safe bowl (with a small amount of water on the bottom) and cook for about 4-5 minutes, until they are tender. Take your olive oil and vinegar and whisk them in a bowl first, then place the rest of your ingredients (along with the white and green beans) together. Stir your liquid in generously so that everything is coated. Serve and enjoy.

Fit Cuisine Notes: 🖊

Serve with grilled chicken or fish of choice and make it a main course. Or make it cold and bring to a friend for a healthy side dish at a BBQ. I made this for Easter dinner one year, and the family loved the fresh taste of this dish.

Time: 20 minutes
Serving: 4-6

Whole Wheat Pasta Salad

WHAT YOU WILL NEED:

1 box whole grain or whole wheat pasta
1 pint cherry tomatoes, chopped
1/2 can of artichokes in water (salad cut)
1 can kidney beans (rinsed)
1 small can black olive (rinsed and chopped)
1 small jar roasted red peppers (rinsed and chopped)
1/2 cup baby carrots, chopped
1 bottle light Italian salad dressing (or olive oil and fresh lemon)

Boil your pasta as the box recommends. In a separate bowl, place the rest of your ingredients, leaving the dressing for last. Once your pasta is cooked, place in the bowl with the rest of your ingredients. Squirt a bit of your dressing on the salad and toss everything together so it's all lightly coated. Place in the refrigerator for about 1/2 hour (if you're strapped for time, you can do all this in advance). Before serving, add a bit more dressing.

FIT CUISINE NOTES: 🖎

This used to be our beach house weekend go-to side dish. It pleases just about everybody's palette. We pair this dish with fish or chicken, or you can just have it as your main meal. Serve at room temperature or chilled. Makes for a great lunch the next day or a showstopper at a BBQ.

Time: 20-25 minutes
Serving: 6-10

Arugula Salad with Slivered Almonds, Diced Apples, Goat Cheese, and Balsamic

WHAT YOU WILL NEED:

1 bag baby arugula
1 apple sliced into matchstick pieces (any apple variety is fine)
1 tbsp slivered almonds
1 tbsp goat cheese crumbles
1 bottle light balsamic vinegar dressing

In a bowl, combine all the ingredients. Toss and serve.

FIT CUISINE NOTES: ✎

I love everything in this salad. I got the idea for it from another one of my favorite places to go in town. The way all the flavors blend in this salad is great—I like to order it as a meal with chicken, scallops, or shrimp. Another great tip is to add fresh lemon if you are not a fan of balsamic vinegar.

Time: 15 minutes
Serving: 4-6

Holiday Sweet Potato Salad

What You Will Need:

2 medium sweet potatoes (1 1/2 pounds), peeled and cut into 1" cubes
1/3 cup nonfat or low-fat plain yogurt
1 small red bell pepper, diced
2 scallions, thinly sliced
3 tbsps chopped, fresh basil
1 tsp red wine vinegar
1/4 tsp salt
1/8 tsp freshly ground black pepper

Place sweet potato chunks in a medium saucepan with cold water filled to just about top. Bring to a boil and cook until tender—8 to 10 minutes. Drain and run under cold water to cool. In a large bowl, combine sweet potatoes, yogurt, bell peppers, scallions, basil, vinegar, salt, and black pepper. Serve at room temperature or chilled.

Fit Cuisine Notes: ✐

This was a dish that I made with my mother. We were getting bored or the traditional sweet potato dishes, so we came up with this lighter version potato salad made with no mayo, butter, or cream. This recipe was great! If you want to impress friends and guest with a different spin on a potato salad this is the one to use.

Time: 40 minutes
Serving: 4-8

Grilled Steak and Vegetable Salad

WHAT YOU WILL NEED:

1 package of lean steak cutlets or sliced flank steak
1 yellow zucchini
1 large tomato
1 asparagus bunch
1 orange pepper, sliced
PAM spray
2 large roasted red peppers (from a jar)
2 tbsps chopped olives (any kind)
1/2 can drained artichokes in water
1 fresh lemon
1 tbsp crumbled goat cheese
2 tbsps light Italian dressing
2 cups arugula salad
1 cup fresh spinach

Marinate your meat with the dressing, and let it sit at room temperature while you get the vegetables prepared. Slice your vegetables so that they cook evenly on your grill, and spray the grill with PAM. Heat should be or medium high, and place *all* your vegetables on top (cook for a total of 10-15 minutes). Place your arugula, spinach, olives, roasted peppers, and artichokes in a large salad bowl. Remove vegetables after they are done—slice them and add to salad bowl. Place steak on grill and cook at same temperature for 5 minutes—but pay attention: they cook really fast!

FIT CUISINE NOTES:

This is a dish inspired by my husband; he is a steak lover. I am not a big fan, but he turned me on to this style of steak. It is lean and, when marinated right, has a lot of flavor. I am a big salad fan; I love putting lots of different vegetables and cheeses into them. So I decided to make us both happy at dinner by mixing the steak and vegetables. It turned out to be a great dish that can be used for a BBQ or lunch the next day. If you really can't do beef, then add shrimp, scallops, or chicken.

Time: 35-40 minutes
Serving: 4-6

Chicken Salad

1-2 cans of white chicken breasts in water, drained (or 4 chicken breasts, poached)
1/2 carrot (shredded using a grater)
1 stalk celery, diced
2 tbsps light mayo
Dash of onion powder
Dash of crushed black pepper

Take your chicken breasts and place them in a bowl. Add your carrots and add celery. Take the mayo and spices and stir together, breaking up the chicken as you like. Let it sit covered in the fridge for 1 hour. Serve.

Fit Cuisine Notes:

I love chicken breasts in a can; they're quick, high in protein, and low in fat. I served this with flat bread I find at Trader Joe's (called Lavasha Bread). It is low in calories and gluten—but 1/2 is a serving, so read the label. You can also put this over mixed greens, or eat as an afternoon snack with whole grain crackers. Clients love this dish, and it's so easy to prepare. It makes for a great lunch the next day or a late-night dinner.

Time: 15-20 minutes
Serving: 4-6

Papaya—Avocado Salad

WHAT YOU WILL NEED:

1 medium papaya, diced
1 medium avocado, diced
3/4 cup jicama, diced
2 tbsps nuts (walnuts, chopped and toasted)
2 tbsps dressing (raspberry vinaigrette, low-fat)

Toss papaya, avocado, jicama, walnuts, and raspberry vinaigrette in a medium bowl. Stir together and serve.

FIT CUISINE NOTES:

This is so refreshing and good. I love all these ingredients. They pair really well on top of fish or chicken, and they can also be eaten with pita chips or whole wheat crackers. I love to put this on top of my mixed greens as a dressing with fresh lemon juice. It is really great cold, and makes an impressive statement at a BBQ.

Time: 10 minutes
Serving: 4-6

Cucumber Roasted Pepper and Tomato Salad

WHAT YOU WILL NEED:

2 large cucumbers (peeled and sliced)
2 large roasted red peppers (from a jar and washed)
1 tbsp sliced black olive (or your favorite type of olive)
6 oz cherry tomatoes, chopped
1 1/2 tbsps cut-up, low-fat mozzarella (slice the block long-ways and cut into small pieces)
Sprinkle of Mrs. Dash (Italian Medley Blend)
1 tbsp plain balsamic vinegar

Take your cucumber, peppers, olives, and tomatoes and put them into a serving bowl. Sprinkle your seasoning on top and toss. Add your balsamic vinegar and cheese, toss again, and serve.

FIT CUISINE NOTES:

This was another dish we ate growing up. I always remember my mother having this salad with dinner in the summer. It has always stayed with me, but I wanted to take a different spin on it by adding a bit more flavor and pizzazz. This was what I felt worked best with these ingredients. You can serve this dish chilled or at room temperature. It's great as a side dish with your favorite grilled protein, or as a refreshing, light salad.

Time: 20 minutes
Serving: 4-6

Spinach and Goat Cheese Salad

WHAT YOU WILL NEED:

1 bag of baby spinach, chopped
2 roasted red peppers, rinsed and chopped
1/4 cup walnuts, chopped
2 cups celery, chopped
1 tbsp oregano
1 tbsp lemon juice
1 tbsp lime juice
1 tbsp extra virgin olive oil
2-3 tbsps goat cheese, crumbled

In a small bowl, mix olive oil, lime juice, lemon juice, and oregano together. Add your spinach, red peppers, and celery together; toss in the liquid mixture. Top with goat cheese and walnuts and serve.

FIT CUISINE NOTES: ✍

This is one of my favorite salads, it has two of my favorite ingredients: spinach and goat cheese. I love the flavor combination of the two, and I started eating spinach salad on a regular basis after discovering I had an iron deficiency. Since I didn't want to eat a lot of meat, I started using vegetables with iron—and spinach is a great one. I love to add shrimp to this salad as a dinner meal or use as a healthy side.

Time: 20 minutes
Serving: 4-6

Pesto Shrimp and Rice Salad

WHAT YOU WILL NEED:

1 cup frozen, cooked shrimp (thawed)
1 package brown rice, cooked
1/3 cup chopped artichokes in water
1/2 cup cherry tomatoes, chopped
2 tbsps olives, chopped
2-3 tbsps fresh pesto (or from the store)
Dash of pepper

Take your shrimp and thaw them under water. Prepare rice as package says. In a sauté pan, heat your shrimp on low with your pesto. Toss the artichokes, tomatoes, and olives, stirring together for no more than 5 minutes. Add your rice and simmer on low for another 5 minutes. Remove from heat and let cool. Serve hot or cold.

FIT CUISINE NOTES:

I love shrimp; it is so good for you and pairs well with just about anything. I made this dish for a BBQ. We needed something that had no meat in it but enough protein—and, of course, plenty of flavor. This dish took no time to make, and it is all prepared in one pot. It was a surprise hit and became a staple on my BBQ menu. If you don't want shrimp, add scallops or chicken.

Time: 20 minutes
Serving: 4-6

Chicken, Tomato, and Broccoli Salad

WHAT YOU WILL NEED:

1 package boneless, skinless chicken breasts
4 cups broccoli florets
1 container grape tomatoes
2 tbsps extra virgin olive oil (divided)
1 tsp sea salt
1 tsp black pepper (freshly ground)
1/2 tsp chili powder
1/4 cup lemon juice

Place chicken in a skillet or saucepan and add enough water to cover. Bring to a simmer over high heat. Cover, reduce heat, and simmer gently until the chicken is cooked through and no longer pink in the middle (about 10-12 min). Transfer to a cutting board. When cool enough to handle, shred with two forks into bite-sized pieces. Bring another large pot of water to a boil, add your broccoli and cook until tender, about 3-5 min. Drain and rinse with cold water. Meanwhile, cut tomatoes in half, crosswise. Do not clean saute pan. Heat the remaining tbsp of oil in the pan over medium heat; along with the tomatoes and chicken. Stir in salt, pepper, and chili powder and cook until fragrant (about 45 seconds). Slowly pour in lemon juice, remove pan from the heat. Toss mixture together and serve.

FIT CUISINE NOTES: ✐

I love this salad. I bring it to a lot of gatherings since I am such a big vegetable fan. It is also a great salad to make for dinner or lunch. It takes no time to prepare, and it is a healthy way to get all your nutrients. I call this the ultimate complete meal. If you don't want to use chicken, just omit the poaching part of the recipe and add tofu, grilled shrimp, or scallops.

Time: 25 minutes
Serving: 4-6

Asparagus with Roasted Almonds

WHAT YOU WILL NEED:

1-3 stalks of asparagus (trimmed)
1-2 tbsps sliced almonds
Olive oil spray

Preheat the oven to 375. Take your stalks, spray them with olive oil, and sprinkle on your almonds. Roast in the oven for about 15 minutes. Remove and serve.

FIT CUISINE NOTES:

I *love* asparagus and eat it every night. This is a great way to jazz up your vegetables and get some added omega 3s from the almonds. Goes great as a side dish with everything, and can be served on any occasion.

Time: 20 Minutes
Serving: 2-4

Whipped Cauliflower

WHAT YOU WILL NEED:

2-3 bags of 16 oz frozen cauliflower (cooked)
2 tbsps olive oil
2-3 tbsps grated parmesan cheese
1/2 cup Italian-seasoned bread crumbs
1 tbsp garlic, minced

Preheat oven to 400. Cook your cauliflower until it's tender, and then drain it. Place your cauliflower in a mixer. Start to add the rest of the ingredients a little at a time and taste as you go. The idea is that you want it to be fully whipped before placing it in the oven. Start by adding a bit of olive oil, then a sprinkle of bread crumbs, then garlic, and then cheese. Mix on medium speed for about 5 minutes. Check the flavors and add whatever you feel is missing from the list above. Once it is at the consistency desired, place into a sprayed casserole dish. Put a little more grated cheese on top and bake until it's almost bubbling on the sides (about 20 minutes).

FIT CUISINE NOTES:

This is a recipe created by my mother, remade by me, and requested by *all* of my clients. The problem with recreating was the measurements. You just need to taste and add all the ingredients above until it's just right. I love its creamy consistency—even though there is no cream in it. I have made this recipe for every occasion, and everyone loves it. I must say, it is a great way to eat a vegetable. Make sure your arms are in good shape prior to making this dish because, if you don't have a mixer, your arms are going to get a good workout!

Time: 30-45 minutes
Serving: 6-8

Whipped Sweet Potatoes

WHAT YOU WILL NEED:

4-6 sweet potatoes (roasted in foils)
Dash of cinnamon
Dash of nutmeg
2 tbsps organic maple syrup
1-2 cups unsweetened Almond Breeze (from the store)

Preheat oven 425. This recipe requires what I call the taste-test-ingredient-adder. Place potatoes on the sheet and bake for 30-40 minutes, depending on the size of your potatoes—they should be soft. Using a mixer (KitchenAid) place the potatoes (skin off), add 1/2 cup of Almond Breeze, 1 tbsp of syrup, and the dashes of cinnamon and nutmeg. Start the blender on a low whip and make sure you get all the lumps out. Taste it; it should be smooth and creamy—if not, repeat the process until you like it. Once you have found the right taste, get a baking dish and spray it with non-stick spray. Place your potato mixture in the dish and sprinkle some cinnamon on top. Bake in the 425 oven for about 10-15 minutes, just so all the ingredients blend together. Take out and serve.

FIT CUISINE NOTES: ✍

This dish was given to me by a friend who has a gluten allergy. I was dealing with a similar issue at the time and he turned me on to this great meal. I had never heard of almond milk before we spoke, but I knew it would taste great in this dish. Let's just say it's a client favorite—I make it every year for Thanksgiving (and for large parties). If you haven't tried almond milk, now is the time—it is low in calories, it has double the amount of calcium compared to regular milk, and it is low on the glycemic index, so it will not spike your insulin levels.

Time: 60 minutes
Serving: 6-8

Roasted Eggplant Spread

WHAT YOU WILL NEED:

1 eggplant
1 tbsp of extra virgin olive oil
1/2 tsp of minced garlic
2-3 celery stalks, chopped
1 red bell pepper, chopped
1 yellow pepper, chopped
2-4 squirts of tomato paste (from a tube or use 1 can)
3 plum tomatoes, chopped
1 cup marinara
2 squirts of pesto (from a tube or 1 tsp from a jar)
Low-fat mozzarella (whole cheese, so you can grate it)
Dash of crushed red pepper flakes
Dash of black peppercorns

Preheat oven to 425. Take your eggplant and shave off only some of the skin (so that it looks like a zebra). Slice your eggplant into cubes and place it on a sprayed baking dish. Place in the oven for about 20 minutes. In a skillet, heat your olive oil and garlic and throw in your celery. Stir until your celery starts to get soft, then add your chopped peppers, tomato paste, and chopped tomatoes. Remove your eggplant from the oven and add to the skillet. Stir in your marinara, crushed red pepper flakes, and peppercorns. Taste to see if the flavors have blended well—if so, add the pesto, stir, and simmer for about 15 minutes. Right before you are ready to plate your spread, take the mozzarella and grate as much as you like into the mixture. Stir and transfer to a bowl.

FIT CUISINE NOTES: ✎

This spread can be served as a main dish by adding whole wheat pasta. You can make it an appetizer with crackers or place it on top of grilled chicken breasts. It tastes even better the next day. This is one of those dishes that has multiple uses.

Time: 30-35 minutes
Serving: 4-8

Sweet Carrots

WHAT YOU WILL NEED:

1 small package baby carrots
1/4 cup water
1 tsp cinnamon
1 tsp butter substitute (Brummell & Brown or Smart Balance)
1 tsp honey

Take all of the ingredients and place them into a small pot. Bring to a boil for about 10 minutes, or until carrots are tender, and serve.

FIT CUISINE NOTES: 🖊

This is a super simple really flavorful side dish that can be made in no time. The kids love this dish as well. I made it for my nieces to try to get them to eat more vegetables with their meals. They loved how sweet and yummy they tasted. A definite must make for the little ones.

Time: 10-15 minutes
Serving: 2-4

Sautéed Green Beans with Cherry Tomatoes

WHAT YOU WILL NEED:

1 (16oz) bag green beans
1 tsp garlic, minced
1 tsp olive oil
1 cup cherry tomatoes, sliced

Place your green beans in a microwave-safe dish for about 5 minutes. Take your beans, oil, and garlic and add them to your sauté pan. Stir together and let cook for about 10 minutes (until tender). Then add your tomatoes and let them get soft for about another 5 minutes. Serve and enjoy.

FIT CUISINE NOTES: ✐

I love green beans, and this is a great way to jazz up a plain vegetable. I have made this dish as a large salad (add another 16 oz bag), a side for the holidays, and a main dish with chicken or shrimp. It can be prepared in no time, and it's filled with nutrients and flavor.

Time: 20 minutes
Serving: 4-6 (If you are making this for a large gathering, just increase the amount of green beans and tomatoes.)

4

HEALTHY AND SIMPLE PASTAS

Baked Whole Wheat Rotini
with Squash

WHAT YOU WILL NEED:

1 box whole grain or whole wheat pasta
1 jar low-salt marinara (or make your own)
1 1/2 cups part-skim ricotta or cottage cheese
2 squirts of pesto
1 large squash, sliced small
1 cup (approximately) shredded mozzarella cheese

Preheat oven to 400. Cook your pasta according to the box. Slice your squash and place it in a baking dish that is sprayed with PAM. Drain your pasta and place it into the dish with your squash, tomato sauce, ricotta, pesto, and shredded mozzarella. Stir the whole thing together so that the flavors blend. Sprinkle some more mozzarella on top and place in the oven for 25 minutes until it's just about golden brown. Remove and serve.

FIT CUISINE NOTES:

This meal is a complete dish. My best friend is crazy about this dish. Though his wife is not a cook, I was able to show her how to prepare this dish. After work, it is her go-to dinner at least once a week. The great thing about this meal is that you can add any vegetable you like. I love the way squash tastes with pasta and marinara, but you can't go wrong with any vegetable.

Time: 40 minutes
Serving: 4-8

Cavatelli with Sautéed Spinach, White Beans, and Cherry Tomatoes

WHAT YOU WILL NEED:

1 bag (1 lb) cavatelli pasta
2 bags (16 oz) chopped frozen spinach (or 4 large bags of fresh spinach)
1 can white beans, drained and rinsed
1 tbsp olive oil
2 tbsps garlic, minced
1 cup cherry tomato, chopped

In a sauté pan, heat up garlic, oil, and spinach. Boil your water for pasta. Sauté the spinach until it's defrosted or wilted. Add your beans and tomatoes and stir them together. Once the pasta is ready, place it into a serving bowl and pour the spinach mixture on top. Toss together and serve.

FIT CUISINE NOTES: ✐

This is a great vegetarian dish. You can use whole wheat cavatelli if you want. I loved this dish as a kid, and it is loaded with iron and fiber. This can be a great side dish when paired with chicken or fish. Add a little Parmesan for extra flavor.

Time: 30 minutes
Serving: 4-8

Elbow Pasta Baked with Vegetables

WHAT YOU WILL NEED:

1 lb elbow pasta (whole grain)
1 lb lean ground beef or ground turkey
1 zucchini diced
1 (28 oz) can crushed tomatoes
1 squash, diced
1 tbsp garlic, minced
1 tbsp olive oil
1 tsp basil
1 tsp oregano
Dash of black pepper
1/2 cup low-moisture mozzarella (optional)

Preheat oven to 400. In a pot, heat up your oil and sauté your garlic and beef. Add your crushed tomatoes and vegetables, and let the entire thing cook until the vegetables are tender and the beef is just about done (the meat is going to continue to cook when you place it in the oven). Cook your pasta a few minutes shy of al dente—the oven will cook it the rest of the way. Drain the pasta and add it to your casserole or baking dish. Take your meat and vegetable pot and pour it on top of the pasta, then mix. Sprinkle the top with the cheese mix one final time. Place it in the oven for about 20-25 minutes. Remove for the oven, let it cool, and serve.

FIT CUISINE NOTES:

This dish is a healthier spin on baked ziti that the kids love. With this dish, you get smaller pasta size, light cheese, and filling vegetables. This is my easy go-to dish if I am doing last-minute entertaining or just looking for a one-pot, complete meal. It can be prepared using the oven or stove top, whichever you prefer.

Time: 30-40 minutes
Serving: 4-8

Spinach, Tomato, and Whole Wheat Pasta

What You Will Need:

1 pound whole-wheat pasta
1 onion or shallot, sliced
1 tbsp extra virgin olive oil
1 (14 oz) can diced tomatoes (drained)
1 pound frozen spinach (or 3 pounds fresh spinach)
Salt and freshly ground pepper, to taste
1/3 cup crumbled feta cheese (or low-fat mozzarella)

Cook pasta according to package directions. Meanwhile, heat oil in a large skillet over medium-high heat and sauté onion or shallot. Add tomatoes; simmer for 10 minutes. Stir in spinach; heat through. Drain the pasta, toss with sauce, and season with salt and pepper. Top with cheese of choice.

Fit Cuisine Notes: 🖊

Yet another fast and healthy meal that uses one pot and cooks up in no time. I love spinach and tomatoes and eat them all the time, so I thought that adding them to a whole grain starch would add extra nutrients and make for a complete dish. What is great about this dish is that you can also add chicken or tofu, serve it hot or cold, and enjoy leftovers the next day.

Time: 30-35 minutes
Serving: 4-6

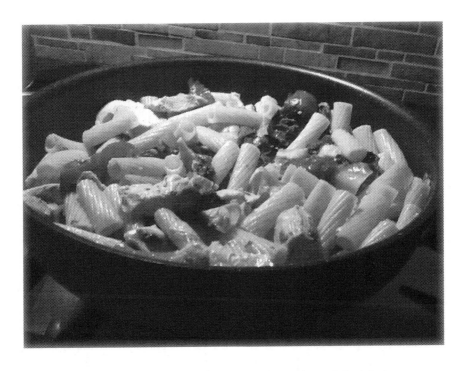

Rigatoni with Sun Dried Tomato, Escarole and Artichokes

Lasagna Rolls

What You Will Need:

1 package whole wheat or regular lasagna noodles
1 medium container part-skim ricotta
1 bag low-fat mozzarella cheese, shredded
1 tbsp Mrs. Dash (Tomato Basil Garlic Blend)
1 jar marinara
1 tbsp olive oil

Preheat oven to 400. Boil water for your noodles (make sure to throw a bit of olive oil into the water so the noodles do not stick). In a bowl, combine about a 1/2 a cup of ricotta, 1/2 cup of shredded cheese, your seasoning, and about 2-3 tbsp of marinara. Drain your noodles and grab a baking dish. Line the bottom of the dish with some sauce. Take an individual noodle and spread your ricotta mixture on top of it, making sure to spread it out evenly. Take one side of the noodle and roll it to meet the other side. Place onto the dish and repeat for each lasagna noodle. Once you are finished, pour the rest of the sauce on top of your lasagna, sprinkle the rest of the shredded cheese on top, and bake for about 25 minutes.

Fit Cuisine Notes:

This is a great way to enjoy the flavors of lasagna without the extra calories or guilt. It is really easy to make, and it can be filled with your favorite vegetable as well. Pair with a large salad and enjoy.

Time: 45-50 minutes
Serving: 6-12

Lemon-Infused Linguine

WHAT YOU WILL NEED:

1 package fresh or boxed linguine
1 cup lemon juice
2/3 cup olive oil
1 tsp Fresh basil, chopped
2 tbsps fresh parmesan

Cook your pasta according to package directions. Once it is cooked, strain it and place into a bowl. Add the rest of the ingredients into your bowl. Toss and serve.

FIT CUISINE NOTES:

This is by far the easiest dish you can make. I love the taste of lemon, and when you add it to fresh pasta and top it with cheese, you have made one impressive dish in a very short amount of time. This can be a great side dish, or you can toss in fresh shrimps and scallops for a full meal.

Time: 20-30 minutes
Serving: 4-8

Escarole with White Beans

What You Will Need:

3-4 heads escarole, chopped and cleaned
1 can cannellini beans, rinsed and drained
5 tbsps water
2 tbsps olive oil
Dash of red pepper flakes
Dash of crushed black pepper

This dish is really healthy and super simple to make. What we are doing here is steaming the escarole first, then adding the rest of the ingredients. This cooks fast, so be prepared. Take your chopped escarole and place it into a sauté pan with your water. Let it start to wilt down on low heat. In a colander, rinse and drain your white beans and set aside. Once the escarole starts to wilt, place your beans, olive oil, and red and black pepper seasonings. Simmer on low, stirring occasionally for about 5 minutes. Serve either like this or with a lean protein of choice.

Fit Cuisine Notes: 🖉

This dish can be paired with a protein, or you can add low-sodium vegetable broth and make it into a soup. Either way, this is a hearty and healthy meal that fills you up without filling you out. This dish was a regular in my house growing up, and I still love making it—especially during the winter months.

Time: 30 minutes
Serving: 4-6

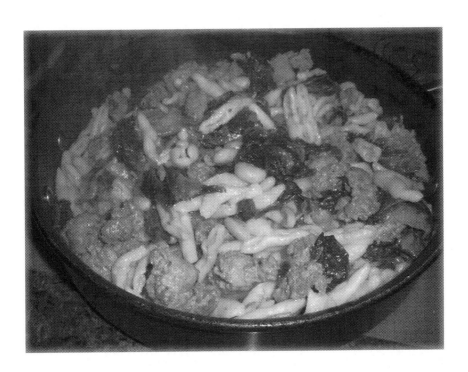

Pasta with Escarole Beans and Turkey Sausage

Roasted Vegetables with Whole Wheat Pasta

What You Will Need:

1 zucchini, sliced
1 squash, sliced
1 bunch asparagus, sliced
1/2 cup butternut squash, diced
1/2 cup broccoli
Nonstick cooking spray (olive oil)
1 (13.5 oz) box whole wheat or whole grain pasta
1 (15 oz) can low sodium diced tomatoes
2 tbsp fresh-grated, low-fat mozzarella
1/2 tsp garlic, minced

Preheat the oven to 400. Slice up all of your vegetables and place them on a sprayed baking sheet. Place in the oven for about 20 minutes. While they are cooking, boil your pasta water. In a large sauté pan, sauté your garlic and tomatoes on low heat. Once the vegetables are done, place them into the sauté pan and heat them up with your tomatoes. Add your cooked pasta and toss it all together so that the flavors can combine. Grate your mozzarella cheese on top of the dish and toss. Serve like that in your sauté pan or transfer to a pasta bowl.

Fit Cuisine Notes:

This is a great dish if you are a vegetarian or if you are just not in the mood for protein. I love roasting my vegetables; it really gives them so much flavor. You can season them with whatever you want and they taste great. This is another complete, quick and healthy meal. If you don't want to use pasta, serve over quinoa or rice.

Time: 30 minutes
Serving: 4-6

Sautéed Zucchini, Eggplant, and White Beans with Whole Wheat Pasta

WHAT YOU WILL NEED:

1 zucchini, sliced
1/2 cup eggplant, diced
1 tsp garlic, minced
1/2 cups small white beans (rinsed)
1 tsp sun-dried tomato pesto
4 cherry tomatoes sliced
Dash of grated parmesan
1 tbsp olive oil
1 (14 oz) box whole wheat or whole grain pasta

Cook pasta according to box. In a sauté pan, heat your garlic and oil. Toss in the zucchini and eggplant. Let the whole mixture cook until the vegetables are tender. Add your cherry tomatoes and pesto, stirring occasionally. By this time, the vegetables should be done and you can toss in the white beans. Heat on medium-low for about 5 minutes, drain the pasta, and pour the mixture over you grains. Sprinkle the parmesan cheese, toss, and serve.

FIT CUISINE NOTES: 🖊

This dish is considered a complete vegetarian meal. I started cooking dishes this way because clients were making requests for meat free meals. In a meat free meal you need protein; beans are the best way to go. They are filled with vitamins and nutrients. The reason you put the beans in last is because they tend to cook really quickly and break apart. If you don't like beans, you can leave them out or add your favorite protein.

Times: 40 minutes
Serving: 4-8

Shrimp and Linguini with Spinach

WHAT YOU WILL NEED:

1 (13 oz) box whole wheat linguini
1 cup shrimp
2-3 cups fresh, chopped spinach
1 tbsp olive oil
1 tbsp garlic, minced
1/2 cup white wine
Dash of pepper
1 tbsp of fresh parmesan cheese

Prepare pasta according to box. In a sauté pan, heat garlic and oil. Add your shrimp and cook for 5 minutes. Toss in drained pasta and spinach, cook for another 5 minutes, add your white wine and pepper. Toss together so all the flavors blend. Remove from heat, top with parmesan cheese, and serve.

FIT CUISINE NOTES: 🖊

This is such an easy and simple dish. I love that everything is prepared in one pot. It is a wholesome meal that can be paired with any protein or vegetable.

Time: 25-30 minutes
Serving: 4-6

Spaghetti Pie

WHAT YOU WILL NEED:

1 box whole grain spaghetti pasta, cooked
2 tbsps olive oil
3-4 tbsps shredded parmesan cheese
1 cup low-fat ricotta cheese
1 cup marinara
1/2 cup low-moisture shredded mozzarella
2 eggs (use an egg substitute)

Preheat the oven to 350. Cook your pasta according to the box, drain well, and toss into a bowl with your olive oil, eggs, and 1 tbsp of parmesan. Grease a pie dish and toss the pasta mixture into the pan, making a nice crust shape out of the noodles. Spoon your ricotta on top along with your marinara. Sprinkle the remaining parmesan on top. Bake in the oven for about 25 minutes, let cool, and serve.

FIT CUISINE NOTES:

My husband always used to talk about how he ate spaghetti pie as a kid. Now he is a big fan of spaghetti. I never heard of this dish (and I'm Italian!), so I decided to research this pie. Here is what I came up with: a complete meal (that can be served with a side salad) made with whole grains and low-fat cheese. My father asked me to make one for him and he loved how it came out as well. Plus, my nieces think they are eating a pizza.

Time: 30-40 minutes
Serving: 4-6

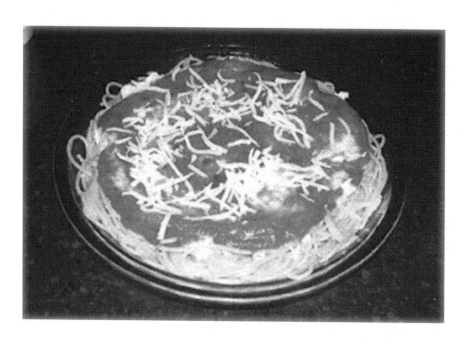

Spaghetti Pie

Low-Fat Spinach Lasagna

WHAT YOU WILL NEED:

1 box lasagna (regular or whole wheat)
1 egg
1 lb low-fat ricotta cheese
1 1/2 cups shredded, low-moisture mozzarella cheese
1 large (16 oz) bag of frozen spinach (drained)
Dash of black pepper and oregano
1 jar tomato sauce (tomato basil or your own creation)

Preheat oven to 375. Cook pasta according to box. In a large bowl, combine ricotta cheese, drained spinach, pepper, oregano, egg, and 1 cup of shredded cheese. Mix together. Drain your noodles. Coat the bottom of a nonstick pan or aluminum baking dish with a ladle of tomato sauce. Layer your noodles and add a small amount of your mixture (spreading it evenly on the pasta) and sauce to the top. Continue this pattern until the noodles are gone. Once finished, add the rest of your sauce and the 1/2 cup of cheese to the top. Cover and place in the oven for 40 minutes, then uncover and continue to bake for another 15 minutes. Once finished, set it aside to cool.

FIT CUISINE NOTES:

This has been my go-to dish for a long time. I make it for all the holidays and prepare it for most of my clients. It is a great way to eat lasagna without eating all that heavy cheese. Plus, you are getting some vegetables in there as well. I have placed this dish in both the fridge and freezer and it reheat beautifully. Now that is what I call an easy make ahead meal.

Time: 40-50 minutes
Serving: 6-8

Stuffed Shells with Zucchini Topping

WHAT YOU WILL NEED:

1 package whole wheat jumbo shells
1 medium container part-skim ricotta
1 small container cottage cheese (1%, low-salt)
3 squirts of tube pesto
2-3 cups marinara
1 zucchini, diced
1 cup shredded mozzarella, low-fat
Sprinkle of black pepper
Sprinkle of Mrs. Dash (Italian Medley Blend)

Preheat oven to 400. Boil your shells according to box. In a bowl, combine 1/2 the container of ricotta with your cottage cheese, pesto, seasoning, and 1/2 cup of sauce. Mix all together. Take your shells and drain them (run under cool water for a second so they are easy to handle). Take your mixture and fill your shells. Place them on a baking dish sprayed with olive oil and filled with some sauce so nothing sticks. Continue filling and placing until shells are done. Pour the rest of your sauce on top of the shells along with your diced zucchini and mozzarella. Bake for about 25 minutes and serve.

FIT CUISINE NOTES:

I made this dish with whole wheat shells, but if you can't find them that's okay. What I love about this dish its satisfying. You can still enjoy your favorite comfort dish without all the unnecessary fat and calories. Since we always need to add vegetables when we can, I decided to dice my favorite veggie, zucchini, and toss that in. Pair well with a large mixed green salad.

Time: 40-50 minutes
Serving: 4-6

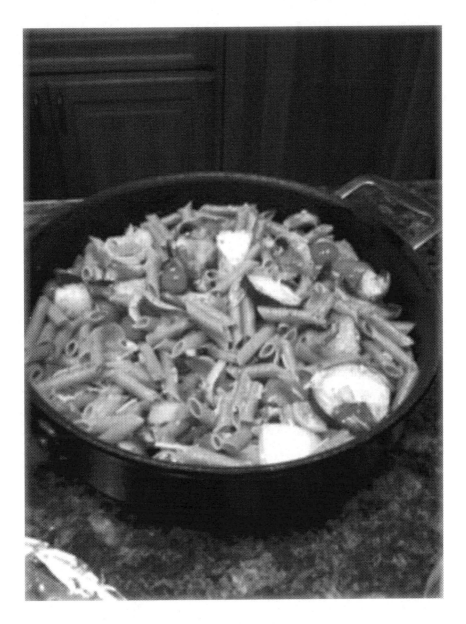

Pasta with Zucchini Squash and tomato

Whole Wheat Baked Ziti

WHAT YOU WILL NEED:

1 box whole grain or whole wheat pasta
1 small container part-skim ricotta
1 tsp basil
1 tsp garlic, minced
1/2 container cottage cheese, lot-fat
1 jar marinara (or your own creation)
1 cup low-moisture shredded mozzarella
1/4 cup parmesan cheese
1 tbsp olive oil

Preheat oven to 400. Cook your pasta according to box. In a pot, throw in your sauce and heat it. In a separate bowl, combine your ricotta, cottage cheese, and basil. Drain your pasta and take out a large baking dish. Put your olive oil and a ladle of your sauce into the bottom of the dish. Pour your pasta into a larger bowl and mix it with your ricotta bowl, adding some more sauce to it. Stir the larger bowl together so that the cheese and pasta stick together. Put the larger bowl into the baking dish, pouring the rest of your sauce on top, along with the mozzarella cheese. Then top with your parmesan. Bake for about 20 minutes, until it starts to become golden brown. Remove from oven and serve.

FIT CUISINE NOTES:

I came up with this recipe for my mother-in-law. She was told by doctors that she needed to stay away from white products, so I made this dish for her during a family gathering. It was great. It had added nutrients from the whole grain and some protein from the cheese. We cut the fat by adding a mixture of cottage cheese and part-skim ricotta.

Time: 20-35 minutes
Serving: 6-8

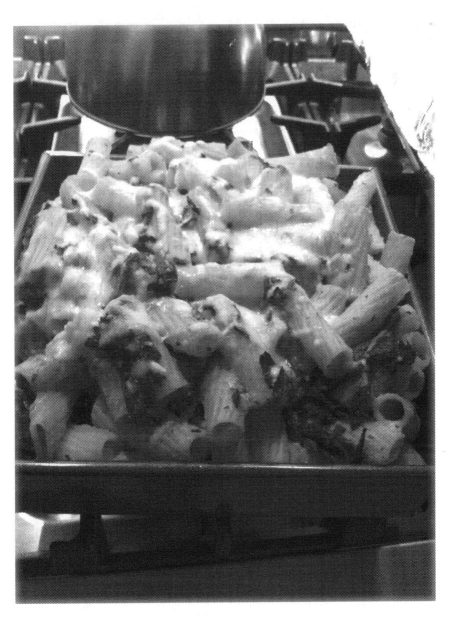

Baked Ziti Fit Cuisine Style

Whole Wheat Orecchiette Pasta with Garlic Oil and Pine Nuts

What You Will Need:

1 box whole wheat or whole grain pasta
1 tbsp toasted pine nuts
1 garlic bulb
2 tbsps olive oil
2 tbsps grated parmesan cheese

Cook pasta according to box. Take your pine nuts and toast them on low heat in a small pot for about 4 minutes. In a sauté pan, heat up your olive oil and garlic bulb. You are not going to mash the garlic; it is going to be infused into the oil (this takes about 5 minutes). Drain your pasta and place into your bowl. Pour the oil and garlic mixture on top and toss together. Add your pine nuts and grated parmesan cheese. Toss again and serve.

Fit Cuisine Notes:

This is a dish that I previewed in one of my cooking classes. It is such an easy and simple dish that can be created with any pasta and paired with any protein you like. I really enjoy the flavors of this dish, and my non-cooking clients who were learning how to make it in class couldn't believe how simple and easy it was. If you want, this dish is a great side for your meals as well. Use whole grain pasta—or regular if you want—and make sure to watch the pine nuts, they cook quickly.

Time: 25 minutes
Serving: 4-8

5

VEGETARIAN AND FISH DISHES

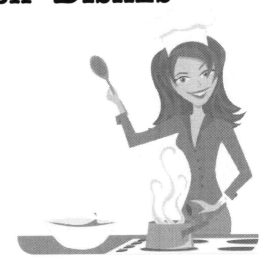

Baked Eggplant Parmesan

What You Will Need:

2 eggplants (sliced lengthwise)
2 egg whites
1 cup panko (Italian-seasoned)
1 jar tomato sauce
1 (15oz) container part-skim ricotta
1 bag low-moisture, shredded mozzarella
2 squirts (or 1 tsp) of pesto
Nonstick cooking spray

Preheat your oven to 425. Make sure your eggplant is sliced lengthwise, no circles. In a small bowl or dish, place your egg whites. In another dish, place your panko. Take a baking dish and spray it with cooking spray. Use your jar of sauce (or your fresh sauce) and cover the bottom of the pan slightly. Take your sliced eggplant and dip it into the egg whites (or brush both sides with egg whites). Then cover with panko and layer the eggplant in the dish. Take your ricotta and place it into a bowl with about 2 tbsps of sauce and your pesto; stir together. Take a few dollops of ricotta and place on different pieces of eggplant (you are not spreading). Sprinkle your shredded mozzarella on top of the ricotta and add a bit more sauce. Then layer your next round of eggplant and repeat the pattern until you are out of ricotta, eggplant, and sauce. Place in the oven for about 30 minutes and serve.

Fit Cuisine Notes:

This is a great dish if you are a fan of eggplant parmesan. It is not fried, so the oil and grease in the dish is pretty much nonexistent. It is very easy to prepare. It tastes better if you let it sit in the refrigerator overnight before cooking. I call this my guilt-free Italian meal. It pairs great with a salad and can be made into a parmesan pita sandwich the next day.

Time: 35-45 minutes
Serving: 4-8

Grilled Vegetable Bake

WHAT YOU WILL NEED:

1 eggplant (cut lengthwise or into circles)
1 yellow squash (cut lengthwise)
1 zucchini (cut lengthwise)
1 fennel bulb (cut into pieces)
1 tomato, sliced
1 small container part-skim ricotta
1 bag part-skim mozzarella
1 jar tomato sauce
1-2 big squirts of pesto (from a tube)

Preheat oven to 400. Take all of your sliced vegetables and place them on your sprayed grill. Make sure they are just about tender before you remove them. In a small bowl, spoon out about 3-4 tbsps of your ricotta. Mix together with your pesto. In a baking dish, ladle some of your tomato sauce to coat the bottom. Place your eggplant on top and spread a bit of your ricotta over the vegetables—you don't want to cover everything, just a bit of each piece. Then sprinkle some of your mozzarella and sauce. Repeat the same pattern for the squash and zucchini (I layer the zucchini and squash together, but you can do whatever you like). Once I get to the top layer, I place the fennel around the sides of the dish and my tomatoes in the middle. Finish it off with another handful of mozzarella and bake covered for about 20 minutes. Remember, the vegetables are already cooked—you are just heating all the other ingredients together so the flavors combine. Once your cheese has melted a bit, remove the lid or foil and bake for another 10 minutes.

FIT CUISINE NOTES: ✐

When I made this dish I prepared it in advance and let it rest. I reheated the dish at 400 degrees for 20 minutes and served it with a side salad. Also, don't be afraid to use a little ricotta—remember, you are not using too much and it is part-skim. I love, love this dish! It uses all of my favorite vegetables, and it takes no time to prepare. If there is a vegetable you are not a fan of, omit it and add whatever you like.

Time: 30-35 minutes
Serving: 4-6

Baked Zucchini Parmesan

WHAT YOU WILL NEED:

6-8 zucchinis, sliced down the middle
1/2 package ground turkey
1 small container part-skim ricotta cheese
2 cups low-moisture, shredded Mozzarella
1/2 jar marinara (or 2 cups fresh)
1 tbsp garlic, minced
2 tbsp olive oil

Preheat oven to 400. Slice your zucchini down the center and set to the side. In a sauté pan, brown your olive oil, garlic, and ground turkey until they are cooked through. In a bowl, place your ricotta, and 4 tbsps of marinara, mixing together. Spray a baking dish with nonstick spray, and coat the bottom with sauce. Start to layer your zucchini like you would lasagna or eggplant. On top of the zucchini, drop a few tsps of your ricotta and turkey (along with the sauce and shredded cheese). You are going to repeat this pattern until you are out of vegetables. Place it in the oven, uncovered, for 25-30 minutes and let it cool for about 5-10 minutes.

FIT CUISINE NOTES: 🗒

This is not fried; it is baked. It is another alternative to eggplant parmesan, using a different vegetable. I served it with a whole grain roll and a salad. You could also serve it with brown rice, quinoa, or whole grain pasta—whatever you like.

Time: 40-50 minutes
Serving: 6-8

Black Bean Burgers

WHAT YOU WILL NEED:

2 (14 oz) cans of black beans, drained and rinsed
1/2 cup whole wheat flour
1/4 cup corn meal
1/2 cup salsa
Dash of cumin

Using a food processor, blend all your ingredients together. Take a baking tray and place parchment paper on it. Using a spoon, roll your bean mixture into balls of any size. Place them on the paper and put the tray in the refrigerator for 1-4 hours. Heat up a grill pan or outdoor grill and flatten your balls out until they are patties. Cook 4-5 minutes on each side. Serve and enjoy.

FIT CUISINE NOTES:

This is a great way to get iron and healthy fiber in your diet. You can make them in advance and leave them in the fridge if you like. The longer they sit in the fridge, the better they taste. Instead of a bun, use a light English muffin. This is a healthy vegetarian dish filled with flavor. Feel free to top with lettuce and tomato—and enjoy.

Time: 35-40 minutes
Serving: 4-6

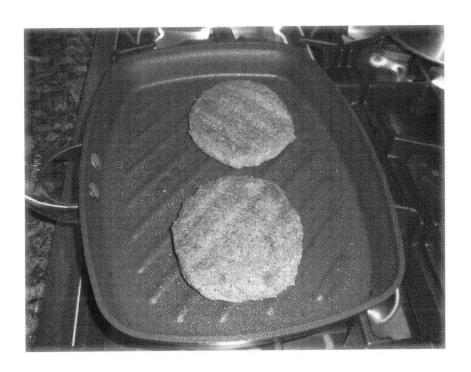

Black Bean Burgers

Easy-Baked Salmon with Fresh Mango Salsa

WHAT YOU WILL NEED:

2-4 salmon fillets
4 tbsps lemon juice (from 2 fresh-squeezed lemons)
1/8th tsp Crushed black peppercorns
1/8th tsp powdered ginger

Salsa (or you can purchase already-made salsa):
1 mango, diced
1 tbsp cilantro, chopped
1/3 cup red onion, finely chopped
1 tbsp lime juice
Pepper to taste

Preheat oven to 400. Coat your salmon with lemon juice, ginger, and black pepper on both sides. Place the fish in the oven and cook for about 15 minutes. While that is cooking, make your salsa. Combine all ingredients in a bowl and stir. Once the fish is done, place your salsa on top and serve.

FIT CUISINE NOTES:

I love Salmon. It is my go-to fish when I am in the mood for seafood. Plus, it is filled with omega-3, which always makes me feel great during my workout the next day. Salmon is one of those fishes that is a bit fishy in taste, but goes great with everything. I am also a big fan of salsa on fish—it's low in calories and sodium and filled with as little or as much flavor as you want. I like mine with mango or pineapple, fairly mild.

Time: 25 minutes
Serving: 2-4

Lemon Pepper Panko Salmon

What You Will Need:

2-4 salmon fillets
2 cups panko bread crumbs
1/3 cup lemon juice
2 tbsps Mrs. Dash (Lemon Pepper Blend)
PAM Baking Spray

Preheat oven to 375. In a dish, place your panko and lemon pepper seasoning and mix together. Take another dish and put your lemon juice into it. Now, with each salmon fillet, dip into the lemon juice first and then the panko (making sure that both sides are coated well). Place on a sprayed baking tray. Once both pieces are done and coated well, put into the oven for 20 minutes and serve.

Fit Cuisine Notes:

Salmon is one of my favorite kinds of fish. It is filled with omega-3 and goes great with everything. I especially love how clean fish tastes with lemon. This dish has the perfect blend of crunch and kick. It pairs well with any vegetable or salad. For an added flavor punch, I love to add 1 tbsp of Greek tzatziki sauce or an avocado.

Time: 25 minutes
Serving: 2-4

Pesto-Topped Grilled Squash

WHAT YOU WILL NEED:

1/2 cup fresh basil, chopped
1/4 cup pine nuts, toasted
1 tbsp extra virgin olive oil
1 tbsp grated parmesan cheese
1 clove garlic, minced
2 tsps lemon juice
1/4 tsp sea salt
2 medium summer squashes (about 1 pound), sliced diagonally
Olive oil cooking spray

Preheat grill to medium-high. Combine basil, pine nuts, oil, parmesan, garlic, lemon juice, and salt in a processor. Coat both sides of your squash slices with cooking spray. Grill the squash slices until browned and tender, 2-3 minutes per side. Remove from grill and spoon your homemade pesto on top and serve.

FIT CUISINE NOTES:

If you don't have time to make homemade pesto, you can use one that is already-made. This is a great side dish, but you can also make it a salad (and add grilled chicken breasts or shrimp to it).

Time: 20-25 minutes
Serving: 4-6

Quinoa and Black Beans

WHAT YOU WILL NEED:

1 tsp canola oil
1 bell pepper, chopped
1 tbsp onion, chopped
1 (15 oz) can black beans, rinsed
1 (8 oz) can low-salt corn
2 tbsps Mrs. Dash (Fiesta Lime Blend)
1/4 tsp cumin
Dash of pepper
2 cups vegetable broth (low-sodium)
1 cup quinoa

Cook up your quinoa using vegetable broth. In a sauté pan, heat up your oil, onions, and peppers until the onions are translucent and the peppers are just about soft. Add your beans, corn, and seasoning, stirring together. Place in a bowl and add your cooked quinoa. Mix together and serve.

FIT CUISINE NOTES:

Make sure to clean the quinoa before cooking. This is a great, slightly spicy dish that is filled with flavor and nutrients. It takes no time to cook, everything is in one pan, and it can be used as a main dish or side at a BBQ gathering. Can be served hot or cold, and it can be saved for lunch the next day.

Time: 30-35 minutes
Serving: 4-6

Ratatouille

WHAT YOU WILL NEED:

1 yellow squash, sliced
1 green zucchini, sliced
1 bunch brussel sprouts, cut in quarters
3 tomatoes on the vine, sliced
2 bunches asparagus, cut
1 cup butternut squash, cut
PAM olive oil spray
Mrs. Dash (Italian Medley Blend)

Preheat oven to 425. Cut up all your vegetables and place on a sprayed baking sheet. Sprinkle them with your seasoning and a bit of olive oil. Make sure all the vegetables are mixed well with the seasoning and bake for 20 minutes. Once finished, toss into a bowl, sprinkle fresh parmesan cheese on top, and serve.

FIT CUISINE NOTES:

I made this dish as a healthy side for Christmas, and it became a regular meal for me during the week. It is so easy and simple to make. I love all the vegetables in this dish, but if there is one you are not a big fan of, you may omit it. You can serve this as a side or a main dish (with beans or meat).

Time: 20-30 minutes
Serving: 4-8

Vegetable and Rice Sauté

WHAT YOU WILL NEED:

1 bag microwavable brown rice
1 zucchini, diced
1 cup broccoli florets
1 squash, diced
1/2 (15 oz) can diced tomatoes with garlic and onion
8 grape tomatoes
1 (10 oz) box of frozen, chopped spinach
1 tbsp olive oil
1/2 cup light Italian dressing
2 tbsps shredded, part-skim mozzarella
5 black olives

Heat up your rice according to package. In a sauté pan, heat up your oil along with all the vegetables (except the spinach). Take your can of tomatoes and place it in your pan along with the oil, grape tomatoes, and spinach. Let the entire dish simmer on low heat until all of the vegetables are soft. Add your Italian dressing and olives, and let it cook for another 5 minutes. Stir together; making sure your spinach is cooked down. Sprinkle your mozzarella cheese on top and serve.

FIT CUISINE NOTES: 🗒

This is one of my husband's favorite side dishes. It takes no time to make, and I created it using leftover, unused vegetables in the fridge and freezer. I served this dish with baked chicken breasts on the side, but you can use shrimp, beef, or your favorite fish if you prefer. It is that simple, and it makes great leftovers.

Time: 20-30 minutes
Serving: 4-6

Whole Grain Pizza Crust

WHAT YOU WILL NEED:

1 (1/4 oz) pack dry active yeast
1 cup warm water
2 cups organic whole wheat flour
1/4 cup wheat germ
Pinch of salt
1 tbsp honey

Preheat oven to 400. In a small bowl, combine your active yeast and warm water, and set it aside so it can get creamy (about 10 minutes). In a separate bowl, combine your 2 cups of flour and wheat germ. Make a well in the middle of the flour and pour your liquid mixture and honey into it. Combine altogether and let sit covered for about 1/2 hour so that it can rise. (You will place your dough on a baking pan and spread it out with your hands.)

FIT CUISINE NOTES:

Since I have a hard time with certain gluten-containing products—yet still love pizza—I wanted to try to find a good solution. So I decided to try whole wheat flour for the first time—and it was good! My husband was not a huge fan but, most times, when I tell him things are healthy, he uses that as an excuse not to *love* it. We ended up having a pizza dough challenge with this recipe—his version versus mine. Let's just say mine tasted the best and left us both feeling good afterward. This is a definite must try for you and your family. Also, use a pizza stone if you have one; it tastes better that way. If not, a baking dish is fine—just spray it with olive oil.

Time: 30 minutes
Serving: 2 small pizzas

Zucchini, Squash, and Tomato Bake

WHAT YOU WILL NEED:

2 zucchini, cut into circles
2 squash, cut into circles
4 tomatoes cut
1 package buffalo mozzarella (part-skim), cut into circles
1 tbsp olive oil
1 shallot, minced
Crushed Pepper
1/4 cup panko bread crumbs
2 tbsps grated parmesan cheese

Preheat Oven to 400. In a sauté pan, cook your shallots in olive oil (about 2-3 minutes). Take a 9" x 9" baking dish, spray it, and place your oil and shallot mixture on the bottom. Take your diced vegetables and cheese and layer them lengthwise in the dish. You should layer them as follows: zucchini, tomato, squash, and cheese. Repeat this pattern until you have used all the vegetables. Next, sprinkle the top with your panko and parmesan cheese.

FIT CUISINE NOTES:

This is a great side dish. It looks beautiful and goes well with just about anything. It can also be made in advance and used as a side dish throughout the week.

Time: 25 minutes
Serving: 4-8

6

SOMETHING-OTHER-THAN-CHICKEN DISHES

Turkey Spinach Meatballs

WHAT YOU WILL NEED:

1 package lean ground turkey meat
1/2 bag fresh baby spinach (steamed)
1 cup tomato sauce (from a jar or fresh)
2 squirts of pesto paste (from a tube)
Sprinkle of Mrs. Dash (Tomato Basil Garlic Blend)
Dash of parmesan cheese

Preheat oven to 400. Take all the above ingredients and mix together. Take small amounts into your hand and form small balls out of the mixture. Place them on a nonstick baking sheet about 1" apart. Place in the oven for 40 minutes and serve.

FIT CUISINE NOTES:

I grew up eating meatballs with pasta every Sunday. I would help my mom make them, place it in the oven until it was ready, and then finish it off with her marinara. To this day, I always bake (never fry) my meatballs, which is healthy tip number one. Number two would be to use lean turkey meat to cut the fat and to add vegetables to the meat for nutrients and extra flavor. This is a great dish that can be served with pasta or as a side with a large salad.

Time: 40 minutes
Serving: 10 meatballs

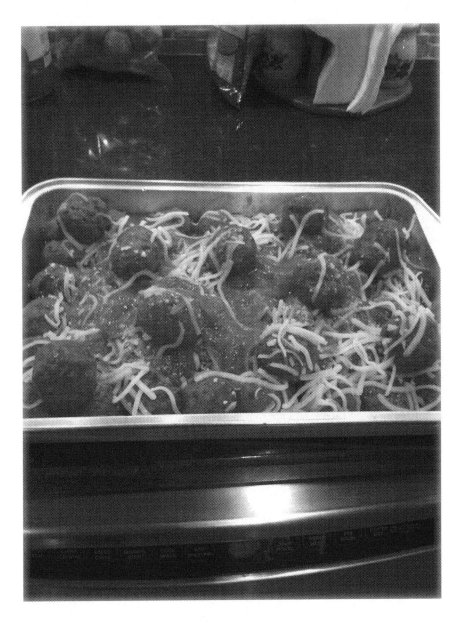

Turkey Meatballs

Spinach and Goat Cheese Turkey Burgers

What You Will Need:

1 package ground turkey
3 oz goat cheese crumbles
1 (10 oz) container frozen spinach (or 1 cup fresh, chopped)
Dash of sea salt
Dash of pepper

Take all your ingredients and mix together. Make your burgers and place on the grill or baking dish. Serve on top of whole grain flat bread, with tomato and your favorite condiments.

Fit Cuisine Notes: 🗒

I like burgers, but I am not a big fan of beef. So, for this dish, I chose ground turkey. I found that, with turkey meat, the flavors are bland, so I added goat cheese and spinach. The flavor combination was insane! Clients enjoy it, and I like preparing it for barbeques. I use flat bread so you don't waste your calories —and it allows you to load up on the tomato and extra spinach if you like.

Time: 30 minutes
Serving: 4-6 portioned patties

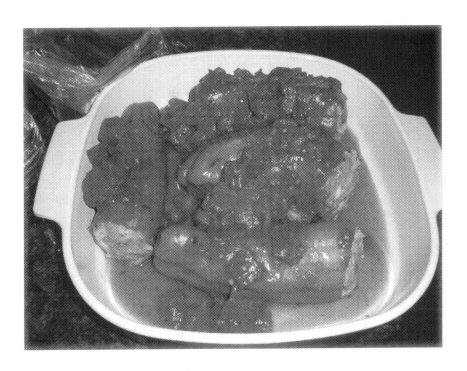

Stuffed Peppers

Italian Turkey Meat Loaf

What You Will Need:

1 package Ground Turkey Meat 93% lean
¼ cup corn flake crumbs
1 tbsp Italian Seasoning
½ cup tomato sauce + ½ cup reserved
2 tbsp Parmesan Cheese

Preheat oven to 425 degrees. In a bowl mix all or your ingredients together. Take a baking dish and coat the bottom with cooking spray. Take your mixture and form it into a loaf. Place in the oven for 40 minutes, remove and pour the rest of your tomato sauce on top. Place back in the oven for another 10 minutes, and serve.

Fit Cuisine Notes:

Meat loaf was a weekly staple in our home growing up. But I started to get board with the traditional ground beef and onion. So I decided to take an Italian spin on this recipe, because who doesn't like the flavors of Italy. The exception to this dish is we are cutting the fat by using lean ground turkey, and instead of traditional breadcrumbs we are used corn flake crumbs. I love serving this with mashed sweet potatoes of a basic side salad and vegetables.

Time: 40-50 minutes
Serving: 4-8

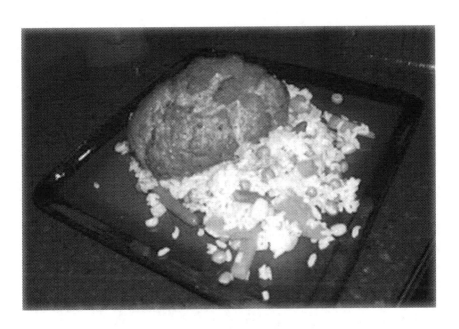

Individual Turkey Meatloaf with Rice

Small Thanksgiving Dinner:

WHAT YOU WILL NEED:

1 Package of Turkey Cutlets
1 Box of whole wheat stuffing
1 small jar or low fat or fat free Turkey Gravy
1 can whole cranberry sauce

Preheat the oven to 375 degrees. In a Ziploc bag place your cutlets and pour half the jar of gravy on top to marinate. Prepare your stuffing according to package. Place your cutlets on a baking dish in the oven for 25 minutes (they cook fast). Take your stuffing and place a little on each dish or your serving dish and put your cutlets on top of the stuffing. Take your cranberries and mash then till soft. Heat up the rest of your jarred gravy, pour it over the cutlets and place the cranberry sauce on top, serve and enjoy.

FIT CUISINE NOTES:

It doesn't have to be a holiday to have traditional food like this. This meal was so fast and flavorful, that I decided I may use this for my own Thanksgiving meal. What is perfect about this dish is portion size; each individual gets a turkey cutlet, some whole wheat stuffing about one scoop, and cranberries. You can't go wrong with that, plus this meal looks like it took forever. Serve with a great side salad.

Time: 30 minutes
Serving 4-6

Stuffed Zucchini Boats

WHAT YOU WILL NEED:

3 zucchinis, sliced in half
1/2 lb ground turkey
3 tbsps quinoa (cooked)
1 tbsp olive oil
2 squirts of pesto (from a tube)
1 cup marinara
3 roasted peppers, chopped (from a jar)
1 small handful baby spinach, chopped
1 handful low-fat mozzarella (shredded)

Preheat the oven to 400. In a sauté pan, heat up your oil and cook the ground turkey, peppers, spinach, and quinoa until the turkey is no longer pink. Add your marinara (use just enough so that the meat is coated) and pesto; stir together. While that is cooking, scoop out your sliced zucchini halves (make sure that you leave some zucchini flesh on the bottom for taste and texture) and place on a sprayed baking sheet. Once the zucchinis are hollow, place your meat mixture inside the boats. Pour 1 tbsp of marinara to the top and then sprinkle some cheese over everything. Place in the oven for about 20 minutes and serve.

FIT CUISINE NOTES:

This dish is one of my clients' favorites, and I get asked to make it all the time. This is a complete meal, filled with flavor. Serve with a salad and enjoy.

Time: 40 Minutes
Serving: 4-6

Stuffed Acorn Squash

What You Will Need:

3 acorn squashes (or match with the number of people you are serving)
1 package sweet turkey sausage links (casing removed)
1/2 tsp garlic, minced
1/2 tsp olive oil
1/2 tsp pesto
4 vine tomatoes (chopped)
1 cup chopped spinach
3 tbsps cooked quinoa
3-4 tbsps marinara

Preheat oven to 400. Take your acorn squashes and slice the tops off, scooping out the seeds and taking the stringy flesh out. Place squashes in the microwave for 3 minutes (until slightly soft). Remove and aside to cool. Take your sauté pan and throw in your olive oil, garlic, and sausage. Let the sausage cook until it is no longer pink. Put your pesto, spinach, quinoa, chopped tomatoes, and marinara into the mixture and stir together over medium heat. Let it blend together for about 5 minutes. Remove pan from heat and place your squash on a sprayed baking tray. Scoop your mixture into the squash and place in the oven for about 20-25 minutes. Remove let them cool for 5 minutes and serve.

Fit Cuisine Notes:

Let's just say that acorn squash does not get the recognition it deserves. You only see it during the holidays, and everyone puts butter and sugar on it. Not a good idea. So I decided to make a complete meal out of one using low-fat ingredients and a lot of flavor. It turned out to be a big hit with one of my clients, and my sister who's not a big vegetable lover. Enjoy with a salad, and show it off to your friends.

Time: 40 minute
Serving: 6-8

Stuffed Peppers with Quinoa

WHAT YOU WILL NEED:

1 lb ground turkey
3-4 peppers (yellow, orange, and red)
4 tbsps cooked quinoa
Small handful baby spinach, chopped
Squirt of pesto (from a tube)
1/4 cup marinara (plus 3-4 tbsps)
6 black olives, chopped
1 tbsp grated parmesan cheese

Preheat oven to 400. Clean the seeds out of the peppers and place the peppers upside down on a sprayed baking sheet for 10 minutes. Remove from oven. In a bowl, combine all the rest of your ingredients and mix well. Take your mixture and place inside your cooled peppers. Place the filled peppers back on the baking dish and add the additional 3-4 tbsps of marinara on top of the peppers. Each one should get about 1 tbsp of sauce. Bake in the oven again for 40 minutes to allow the stuffing to be cooked completely. Remove cool for 5 minutes before serving.

FIT CUISINE NOTES:

My mom is known for making *great* stuffed peppers. She makes them all the time. Growing up, we always had them. As I got more involved with healthier eating, however, I needed to find a way to make the family staples on my own terms. So, with my peppers, I omit the green (too hard to digest) and, instead of using rice and ground beef as a binder (which my mom uses), I use quinoa. I find that using rice and beef makes the dish too heavy. My ingredients make it clean and light. Clients enjoy it, it takes no time to make, and you get all your nutritional components in one dish. Serve with a mixed green salad and enjoy.

Time: 45-50 minutes
Serving: 3-4 (depending on the amount of people preparing for)

Pork Stir-Fry with Noodles

WHAT YOU WILL NEED:

6 oz whole grain spaghetti cooked
1 package mixed vegetables of your choice, frozen
1/2 cup teriyaki sauce
Fresh lemon rind
Dash of ginger
1 package pork tenders
1 tbsp vegetable oil

Cook your pasta according to package. In a sauté pan, heat up your oil and throw in your pork. Cook through before adding your package of mixed vegetables, lemon, and ginger. Cook on medium-low heat for about 5 minutes. Add your pasta and sauce, stir together, and let simmer for another 10 minutes. Cool and serve.

FIT CUISINE NOTES: 🖊

This is a great, well-rounded, complete meal. It is even better the next day. If you are not a fan of pork, you can use chicken or shrimp. Make sure to read the sodium label on the teriyaki sauce—look for a low-sodium version of your favorite brand.

Time: 30 minutes
Serving: 2-4

Marinated Italian Pork Loin

WHAT YOU WILL NEED:

1 large pork tenderloin
1 bottle light Italian dressing
1 tbsp parmesan cheese
1 tsp Mrs. Dash (Italian Medley Blend)

Take a Ziplock bag and place all your ingredients in it. Seal and massage dressing into the meat. Refrigerate for 30 minutes or overnight. Preheat oven to 400. Put the pork and all the juices into a baking dish and cook for 40 minutes (or until pork is not too pink). Serve and enjoy.

FIT CUISINE NOTES:

This is by far the quickest and easiest meal you can prepare. If you are a pork lover, then this dish is for you. It can be prepared overnight so it's ready to go the next day. Pork is considered the other white meat because it is so lean, especially tenderloins. Serve with a great vegetable or salad, and use the extra pieces for lunch the next day.

Time: 40-45 minute
Serving: 4-8

Low-Fat Turkey Bolognese

What You Will Need:

1-2 lb package lean ground turkey breast
1 cup carrots, chopped
1 cup celery, chopped
1 shallot, chopped
1 tbsp garlic, minced
1 tbsp extra virgin olive oil
2 (15.5oz) cans diced tomatoes
1 1/2 jars tomato basil sauce (your favorite brand)
1 lb whole wheat or whole grain pasta
Dash of oregano
Dash of basil
1 (8oz) can olives, chopped (optional)

In a large pot, heat oil and add your garlic, shallots, carrots, and celery. Cook them until they are just about tender. Next, add your ground turkey and cook it until it is no longer pink. Once your turkey is cooked, add your diced tomatoes and tomato basil sauce. Get your pasta water ready to cook; follow package directions. Let the sauce come to a boil and then simmer for about 20 minutes (until vegetable are soft). Add your spices and stir occasionally so that all the flavors can infuse. Once the pasta is done, drain and place it into your pasta bowl. Ladle as much of the Bolognese onto the pasta as you like, and toss in your olives (if you are going to use them). Serve with fresh parmesan cheese and enjoy.

Fit Cuisine Notes: ✐

This is my all-time favorite go-to dish for all occasions: anything from a weeknight dinner with my husband to a last-minute visit with family and friends. You cannot go wrong with this recipe; it tastes great with or without pasta. If you wanted to change the flavor of the dish, you could omit the celery and carrots and add zucchini and squash. We love it!

Time: 30 minutes
Serving: 4-8

Crusted Pork Loin with Tomato

WHAT YOU WILL NEED:

1 large pork tenderloin
1/2 cup cornflake crumbs
1/2 cup Italian-seasoned panko
1 tbsp Mrs. Dash (Italian Medley Blend)
Nonstick cooking spray
1 can fire-roasted tomatoes
1/4 cup low-calorie Italian dressing

Preheat oven to 400. In a Ziploc bag, place your pork and dressing. Shake it around so everything is nicely coated. Remove your pork from the bag and place it on your baking dish. Season each side with your Italian seasoning, and then coat each side of your pork with the cornflake crumbs and panko. Make sure that all the pork is covered well and top with your canned tomatoes. Place the entire baking dish into the oven for about 45 minutes—or until meat is no longer pink. Serve in slices and enjoy.

FIT CUISINE NOTES:

I decided to cook this dish for my husband in the middle of the week. He loves pork, but tenderloin is a very lean cut, so it needs to be flavored well. I was starting to get bored with the same honey mustard or soy sauce marinades. So I decided to encrust it with cornflakes and panko. It was *awesome!* I also topped it with fire-roasted, diced tomato to add a bit of a kick. This is a must try. I served it over whole grain pasta with roasted broccoli. It's a quick, mid-week surprise for your loved ones, and it doubles as lunch for the next day.

Time: 45-60 minutes
Serving: 4-6

Chicken Sausage Ragout

WHAT YOU WILL NEED:

1 package chicken sausage, diced
1 zucchini, diced
1 squash, diced
1 can white beans (rinsed and drained)
1 (16oz) bag frozen, chopped kale
2 cans low-salt, diced tomato
Dash of pepper
3 cups low-sodium chicken broth
1 tbsp garlic, minced
2 tbsps olive oil

In a medium pot, sauté your oil and garlic. Add your zucchini, squash, and sausage, and let that cook for 5 minutes. Then add your chicken broth, kale, and diced tomatoes, let it simmer for 10 minutes. At this point, the sausage is nearly cooked and your vegetables are tender. Add your beans and pepper. Stir together and let it simmer on low for 5 minutes. Remove from heat and serve.

FIT CUISINE NOTES:

This was the first time I ever cooked with kale. I normally use spinach (which can be used instead), but I was bored and wanted to try something different. Since kale is known for its nutritional benefits, I thought, why not? I must admit that I really like the way it turned out. The slightly bitter taste went really well with the sausage kick. Plus, everything was made in one pot, which made it quick and easy. To give it just a little more flavor, I sprinkled parmesan cheese on top before serving. I would not add a starch to this dish since it is made with beans.

Time: 30-35 minutes
Serving: 4-6

Brown Rice Bake with Meatballs

WHAT YOU WILL NEED:

Baby turkey meatballs: look at past recipe for meatballs
1 bag instant brown rice (or microwavable brown rice)
1/2 cup part-skim mozzarella
2-3 tbsps parmesan cheese
1 (15 oz) can diced tomato (no salt)
1/4 cup of marinara (light)

Preheat oven to 375. In a bowl, combine your cooked rice, mozzarella, tomato sauce, and diced tomatoes. Stir the whole mixture together and throw it into a baking dish. Place your meatballs (cooked) on top and sprinkle everything with your parmesan cheese. Place in the oven for about 10-15 minutes and serve. Note: you can also purchase your meatballs in the health foods frozen section. A normal serving is 3, but that can be doubled for larger families.

FIT CUISINE NOTES:

This was a favorite of mine when I was a kid. My mom used to make this with ground meat and, of course, white rice. But I wanted to make it healthier. I would absolutely recommend making this dish with vegetables. You could add chopped spinach or squash (both are really flavorful and would make this a quick, complete meal). The kids will enjoy this as well.

Time: 30 minutes
Serving: 4-6

Healthy Sausage and Peppers with Brown Rice

WHAT YOU WILL NEED:

1 Package of Chicken Sausage (Italian Style)
2 Red Peppers (diced)
2 Yellow Peppers (diced)
2 Orange Peppers (diced)
1 package or brown rice (Uncle Ben's Instant) or Microwave rice packets
2 1/2 cups of your favorite Tomato Basil Sauce or Fresh
1 tsp Parmesan cheese
1 hand full of Low Fat Mozzarella

Preheat oven to 400 degrees. Take your rice and cook it as the package says. Chop up your vegetable fine and add them to your cooked rice in a large bowl and mix together. Either dice your sausage or leave it whole, I prefer to dice. Mix the remaining ingredients in the bowl, (sauce, cheese). Pour the entire mixture into a sprayed baking dish and sprinkle the top with your low fat mozzarella, and the bit more sauce. Bake in the oven for about 30 minutes. Let cool and serve.

FIT CUISINE NOTES: ✎

This is a great dish for pot luck dinner, BBQ's or parties. It is a great healthy twist on your traditional sausage and peppers. I love to use chicken sausage as well, it is hormone free, gluten free and is full of flavor, plus they come in a variety of seasoning. This is a great one pot meal that can be made over the weekend, freeze and have during the week, or you can prepare it the night before or morning of let it sit in the refrigerator and cook later on. Either way you can't go wrong with this recipe.

Time: 30-40 minutes
Serving: 4-8

7

ENDLESS CHICKEN DISHES

Quinoa with Spinach, Chicken, and Feta Cheese

WHAT YOU WILL NEED:

1 cup uncooked quinoa
2 cups water
1 tbsp olive oil
2 whole garlic cloves
4 cups fresh spinach (or 16 oz frozen bag, water drained)
1 ounce reduced-fat feta crumbles
1 package chicken tenders, diced

Follow the cooking directions on your quinoa. In a sauté pan, place your olive oil and garlic. Cook on medium-low heat until the garlic is brown. Once brown, remove from the oil and set aside. We are infusing the oil here—we don't want an overpowering taste. Then throw in your diced chicken and cook thoroughly. Once it is just about done, add your spinach and let it cook down slightly (about 5 minutes). Remove your cooked quinoa and toss it into a bowl (or put into a serving platter). Pour your sauté pan mixture over the quinoa and sprinkle with your crumbled feta.

FIT CUISINE NOTES:

I had this recipe published in July's 2011 issue of Bella Magazine. It is a great, complete, low-starch meal. I love using quinoa, but if you are not a fan you can use whole grain pasta or rice. It tastes great hot or cold, and it can even be used as a salad.

Time: 25-35 minutes
Serving: 4

Rotisserie Chicken and Fresh Vegetable Bake

What You Will Need:

1 roasted chicken, diced
1 bunch asparagus, diced
1/2 eggplant, diced
1 yellow squash, diced
1 cup green beans (fresh or frozen)
1 jar marinara
1 can low-sodium, diced tomato
1 cup shredded, low-fat mozzarella
2 tbsps Mrs. Dash (Tomato Basil Garlic Blend)
2-3 squirts of pesto (from a tube)

Preheat oven to 400. In a large baking dish, place your diced tomatoes. Then just start tossing all your vegetables and chicken together. This dish has no sequence, but make sure that you put a bit of marinara in between all the food layers. Once you have put everything together, squirt your pesto, add some more marinara, and mix together while in the baking dish. Sprinkle with your cheese and place in the oven for about 20 minutes (until the vegetables are soft and tender).

Fit Cuisine Notes: ✍

I use this recipe at least once—maybe even twice—a week. It is my quick, go-to healthy meal that can be paired with just about any vegetable or grain you like. What I do is purchase a Perdue Rotisserie Chicken in a bag and bake it over the weekend. Then I slice it, place it in a container, and serve it during the week. If you don't want to make one, then buy one you like. This is a great, one-dish, complete meal that makes plenty of leftovers.

Time: 30 minutes
Serving: 4-8

Spaghetti Squash with Chicken, Zucchini, Sun-Dried Tomatoes, and String Beans

WHAT YOU WILL NEED:

1/2 spaghetti squash (cooked)
1 package chicken breasts, diced
1 zucchini, diced
1 small bag French-cut green beans (defrosted or fresh)
2 cups marinara
1 forkful sun-dried tomatoes, julienne
1 tbsp olive oil
1/2 tsp garlic, minced
Small handful low-fat mozzarella cheese

Preheat the oven to 425 and slice your spaghetti squash in half. Place on a sprayed baking dish, skin-side up, and put into the oven for 40 minutes. In a skillet, heat your olive oil and garlic and throw in your diced chicken. Cook your chicken until it's no longer pink. Add your green beans, zucchini, and marinara. Cook until the zucchini and the beans are tender. Remove your spaghetti squash from the oven and let it cool for about 15 minutes. While it is cooling, simmer your skillet for the same amount of time. Take a fork and scrap the spaghetti squash out of the skin and throw it into your skillet. Toss altogether and add your sun-dried tomatoes and mozzarella.

FIT CUISINE NOTES: 🗒

This is a great, low-carbohydrate meal. If you have not tried spaghetti squash (or have no idea how to cook it), let me be the first to tell you that it is really easy and very tasty—as long as you follow my simple steps. With this dish, if you don't like chicken you can always make substitutions or omit the meat altogether. My suggestion is to get your squash, cook it over the weekend, and place it in the refrigerator to use during the week. This way, you always know it's ready to go. This will cut your cooking time in half.

Time: 45-50 minutes
Serving: 6-10 (depending on the size of the squash)

Pesto Baked Chicken
with Roasted Peppers

What You Will Need:

1 package chicken breasts
2 tbsps olive oil
2-3 squirts of pesto (from a tube, or 1 tbsp from a jar)
2 tbsps grated parmesan cheese
1/2 cup panko bread crumbs
1/2 cup cornflake crumbs
4 slices roasted red peppers (rinsed)

Preheat Oven to 400. In a Ziploc bag, place your chicken, panko, cornflakes, olive oil, pesto, and grated cheese. Close the bag and mix all of the ingredients together until all parts are coated. Place the chicken on a sprayed baking sheet and place a roasted pepper on top of each piece of chicken. Bake in the oven for about 20-25 minutes, depending on the thickness of your chicken. Serve and enjoy.

Fit Cuisine Notes:

This is a great way to enjoy baked chicken. This was the first time I used cornflakes, and it gave the chicken a little added sweetness and crunch—especially when paired with the panko. If you are not a fan of the cornflakes, then use panko or regular breadcrumbs (with Italian seasoning). Serve alongside a salad or vegetables and enjoy.

Time: 30-40 minutes
Serving: 4-6

Baked Chicken Parmesan

WHAT YOU WILL NEED:

1 package chicken breasts
1-2 tbsps Mrs. Dash (Italian Medley Blend, no salt)
2 tbsps olive oil
1 cup panko bread crumbs (plain)
1/2 jar light tomato sauce (or fresh)
1 cup low-fat mozzarella cheese

Preheat oven to 400. In a Ziploc bag, place your seasoning, panko, and chicken. Seal well and shake it up so all the pieces get completely covered. Remove the chicken from the bag and place in a sprayed baking dish. Pour your 1/2 jar of tomato sauce over the chicken and sprinkle with mozzarella. Place the dish in the oven for about 30-35 minutes, until the chicken is cooked. Once done, you can sprinkle with a little more cheese (if you desire) before serving.

FIT CUISINE NOTES:

This is the first time I used panko. Panko is great—you can buy them with Italian seasoning or plain (like I did) and add your own seasoning to avoid extra salt. It tastes great and it's made with half the fat because you are not frying it first. Pairs really well with a salad, steamed vegetables, or whole grain pasta. Just another decadent traditional meal without extra fat and calories.

Time: 30-40 minutes
Serving: 4-6

Broccoli, Chicken, and Rice Bake

WHAT YOU WILL NEED:

1 package chicken breasts
1 can cream of broccoli soup (low-sodium)
1 cup unsweetened almond milk (or low-fat milk or water)
1 cup fresh, chopped broccoli
Dash of paprika
Dash of black pepper
1 cup brown rice or orzo (uncooked)

Preheat oven to 400. Take a casserole dish and throw in the contents of your soup can, milk, paprika, pepper, and chicken. Top with your rice and broccoli, mix in the liquid, and place (covered) in the oven for about 40 minutes. Serve and enjoy.

FIT CUISINE NOTES:

It doesn't get any easier than this recipe. This is one of those recipes for which you can't use the I-have-no-time-to-cook excuse. I prepared this dish in the morning while sipping coffee before work. I let it sit uncooked in the refrigerator so that, when I got home from my long day, all I needed to do was turn the oven on and let it cook. This is a full, one-dish meal that includes all food groups.

Time: 40 minutes
Serving: 4-6

Balsamic Chicken with Mushrooms, Tomatoes, Olives, Basil, and Goat Cheese

What You Will Need:

1 bag portion-controlled chicken breasts (Perdue, for example, has 4-6 per bag)
1 tsp Mrs. Dash (Tomato Basil Garlic Blend, no salt)
1/2 cup balsamic vinegar
1/2 container mushrooms, chopped
1/2 pint cherry tomatoes, diced
2-3 tbsps olives, sliced
1 tbsp fresh basil
1 tbsp crumbled goat cheese
1 tbsp olive oil or PAM spray

On a cutting board, season your chicken with Mrs. Dash. Heat a nonstick skillet with olive oil spray, place your chicken in the skillet, and cook it on both sides. Place your chopped mushrooms, tomatoes, and olives in a bowl. Remove your chicken and set it to the side. Pour your balsamic vinegar into the skillet with all the leftover chicken juices. Add the chicken back in with your vegetables. If you find it needs more balsamic, now is the time to add it. Turn the heat down to low, and let it simmer for 5 minutes. Put the chicken on a plate and add the balsamic sauce on top. Sprinkle with the basil and goat cheese and serve.

Fit Cuisine Notes:

If you don't like mushrooms, use squash or green beans. This dish is a great twist on plain balsamic chicken. It's great for entertaining. I actually made this for a cooking party I hosted, and the guest loved it. You can serve it with a side salad or on a bed of quinoa, rice, or whole grain noodles.

Time: 30 Minutes
Serving: 4-6

Grilled Chicken Greek Salad

WHAT YOU WILL NEED:

4 chicken breasts
1 tbsp lemon juice
1 tbsp olive oil
1 tbsp oregano, fresh (or 1 tsp dried)
2 cloves garlic, minced
1/4 tsp black ground pepper
3 medium cucumbers, seeded and coarsely chopped
2 medium tomatoes (red or yellow), coarsely chopped
1/2 cup red onions
Lettuce, sliced (mixed greens)
1/3 cup dressing (reduced-calorie creamy cucumber)
1/2 cup crumbled feta cheese
1/4 cup kalamata olives (pitted)

Place chicken in a shallow dish. For your marinade, in a small bowl, combine lemon juice, oil, oregano, garlic, and pepper. Pour over chicken. Turn to coat chicken and marinate in the refrigerator for a few hours. Meanwhile, in a medium bowl, toss together cucumbers, tomatoes, and red onion. Drain chicken and discard your marinade. Place chicken on the rack of an uncovered grill, directly over medium coals. Grill for 12-15 minutes (or until tender and no longer pink), turning once. Remove from the grill and let it sit for a few minutes so the juices can rest. Slice the chicken into strips and place on top of the salad. Toss your feta and olives on top of the salad and serve.

FIT CUISINE NOTES:

This is a great, complete salad. It is filled with light flavors that everyone will enjoy. This happened to be my mother's favorite dish. If you are not a fan of chicken, you can use beef or shrimp. And if feta is not on the top of your list of cheeses, use mozzarella—it is just as flavorful.

Time: 30-35 minutes
Serving: 4-6

Chicken Breasts Stack with Mozzarella and Tomato

What You Will Need:

1 package chicken breasts
1 small container (3 oz) fresh mozzarella, sliced
2 fresh tomatoes
3-4 tbsps balsamic vinegar
1 tbsp Mrs. Dash (Italian Medley Blend)

Preheat the oven to 375. Place your balsamic and your Italian seasoning into a bowl and stir together. Place your chicken on a baking dish and brush with your now-prepared marinade. Place in the oven and bake for 15 minutes. Then remove from the oven, add your mozzarella and tomato to the chicken, and put it back in the oven for another 15 minutes. Remove and let cool. Serve on top of rice, noodles, or with a salad and vegetables.

Fit Cuisine Notes: ✎

This is like a non breaded chicken parmesan. I wanted a way to get a low-calorie, portioned-out dish that had the flavors of the traditional dish without the extra sauce and cheese. So I thought about layering the ingredients and seeing how it turned out. Well, it was great!

Time: 30-40 minutes
Serving: 4-6

Chicken Roll-Up with Goat Cheese and Asparagus

WHAT YOU WILL NEED:

4 thin chicken breasts
1 small roll herb goat cheese
5 tbsps balsamic vinegar
1 tbsp olive oil
1 tsp Mrs. Dash (Tomato Basil Garlic Blend, salt-free)
8 asparagus spears cut in half

Preheat the oven to 400. In a small bowl, combine your balsamic vinegar, olive oil, and seasoning. Stir together. Take your chicken breasts and place them flat on the cutting board. Use your goat cheese roll to spread a layer along the top of the breast. Take 2 spears of asparagus and place them on the top of the chicken. Slowly start to roll the chicken breasts down to the other end, wrapping the spear up with it. Take a sprayed baking dish and add your chicken. Use your balsamic marinade to coat the top and sides of the chicken with a brush, making sure you get everything coated. Place in the oven and bake for about 25 minutes. Remove from oven and serve.

FIT CUISINE NOTES:

I love asparagus; I eat it just about every night. With this recipe, I wanted a fun way to eat asparagus using a protein. So, I decided that, instead of dicing up the chicken and asparagus and making the dish the same way I always did, why not wrap the chicken around the vegetable and use the cheese as my flavor-binding agent inside. So I tried it and, although it looked funny, it tasted amazing. If you are not a big fan of goat cheese, try gruyere or low-fat mozzarella. Serve alongside a baked sweet potato, quinoa, or a salad.

Time: 30-40 minutes
Serving: 4-6

Chicken with Mango and Peach Salsa

WHAT YOU WILL NEED:

2 tbsps olive oil
1 package chicken breasts (skinless)
1 small jar mango, peach, or pineapple salsa (Newman's is really good)
1 package or 1/2 cup of brown rice

Place oil in a nonstick skillet and heat for about 1 minute. Place your chicken breasts in the pan and let them cook until they're no longer pink (you may need to flip them once or twice). About 10 minutes into the cooking process, place 3 tbsps of the mango salsa (or whatever salsa you found) on top of the chicken and let it simmer. While that is cooking, prepare your rice (according to the package). Pour the rest of the salsa over the chicken; let it simmer for another 5 minutes, and serve.

FIT CUISINE NOTES:

I love to serve this with brown rice, and ladle the chicken mixture over it. This way, you can taste all the flavors in one bite. Include a nice side salad or vegetable and you are good to go.

Time: 30 minutes
Serving: 4-6

Stuffed Chicken with Spinach, Roasted Red Peppers, and Mozzarella

What You Will Need:

1 package chicken breasts
4-6 oz balsamic vinegar
1 tsp Mrs. Dash (Tomato Basil Garlic Blend)
Dash of grated parmesan cheese
1 small bag baby spinach
1 small jar roasted red peppers (rinsed)
Fresh, part-skim mozzarella cheese (Polly O), sliced

Preheat oven to 400. Take your chicken breasts and slice them, butterfly style (not all the way through). Take your chicken and place it in a Ziploc bag. Using a mallet or a frying pan, pound the chicken breasts until they are thin. In a small bowl, combine your vinegar, seasoning, and cheese. Stir together. Take a basting brush and coat your pounded, butterflied chicken. Stack a few pieces of baby spinach, a small slice of roasted pepper, and your mozzarella on one side of your chicken. Fold the other half of the chicken and close it up (if you want, you can seal it with a toothpick). Place your stuffed chickens on a PAM sprayed baking dish. If you have more dressing, coat the rest of the pieces and bake.

Fit Cuisine Notes:

I love stuffed chicken; it is filled with so much flavors. When you order it in a restaurant, it is usually loaded with oil, cheese, and, sometimes, butter. I decided to try my own version using my favorite combination of flavors and texture. It goes really on a bed of whole wheat linguini.

Time: 30 minutes
Serving: 4-6

Broccoli and Chicken Pie

WHAT YOU WILL NEED:

2 cups fresh broccoli florets, steamed (or a 12 oz thawed, chopped bag)
1-2 cooked chicken breasts, diced
1/2 cup low-fat cheddar cheese (1/4 cup reserved)
1/3 cup cherry tomatoes, sliced
1/2 cup Original Bisquick mix
1 cup fat-free milk
2 eggs (use an egg substitute)
1/4 tsp black pepper

Preheat the oven to 400. Spray a 9" pie dish with PAM. Put the broccoli, tomato, and chicken into your dish. Sprinkle with 1/2 cup of cheese. Next, mix up your Bisquick, eggs, milk, and pepper so that it is not lumpy. Pour the mixture into the dish and place it in your oven for about 30-35 minutes. Remove from the oven and sprinkle the dish with the rest of your cheese. Put the dish back in the oven to bake for another 5 minutes. Serve and enjoy.

FIT CUISINE NOTES: ✐

I have to say that I am a bit obsessed with these pies. I was inspired by watching a chef on a cooking program make frittatas, but I was not into all the creams and cheeses that went into them (and they took forever to make). I needed something I could make in one dish that could be made quickly after work. So I decided to try one with Bisquick. I had seen the pictures on the boxes, so I wanted to give it a try—adding my own healthy ingredients to save time and calories. I loved the way this came out, so I developed other pies using a variety of vegetables. This recipe can even be used entertaining a brunch or yourself the next day, just reheat and enjoy.

Time: 30-35 minutes
Serving: 6-8

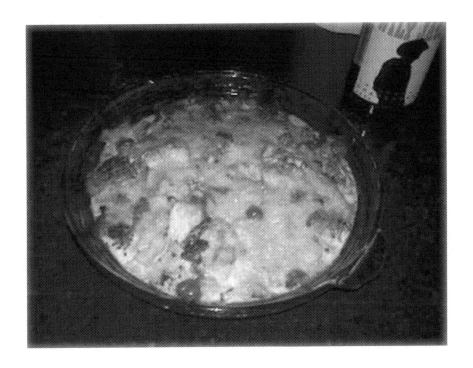

Broccoli Pie

Chicken Breasts with Roasted Red Peppers, Artichokes, and Sun-Dried Tomatoes

What You Will Need:

4 tbsp balsamic vinegar
1 package chicken breasts
1 medium jar roasted red peppers
1 (8 oz) jar artichoke hearts (with oil)
1 (8.5 oz) jar sun-dried tomatoes, julienned in olive oil

Preheat oven to 400. Coat the bottom of a medium-size pan with balsamic vinegar. Take your package of chicken and place it in the pan (if the chicken is too thick, you can slice the breasts down the center to make them thinner). On top of each piece of chicken, add a layer of roasted peppers, artichokes, and sun-dried tomatoes. Continue until the jars are empty and all pieces of chicken are nicely coated. Place in the oven for about 30-40 minutes (or until chicken is cooked all the way through).

Fit Cuisine Notes: ✑

My husband loves this recipe. I have made it so many times with so many different ingredients. It is great to bring to potluck dinners or to serve to the family (and have leftovers for lunch). If you want, you can serve it with brown rice or whole grain pasta—or you can just serve it with a simple side vegetable or salad. Enjoy!

Time: 30-40 Minutes
Servings: 4-6

8

HEALTHY AND SIMPLE
ALMOST-DESSERTS

Piña Colada Cake

WHAT YOU WILL NEED:

1/2 cup toasted coconut
1 box white cake mix (with the pudding included in the mix)
1/2 cup water
1/2 cup 100% natural pineapple juice
1/3 cup light Bacardi rum
4 egg whites
1 can pineapple filling (Whole Foods)

Simple Syrup:
1/2 cup pineapple juice 100% Natural
1/2 cup sugar

Frosting:
2 containers vanilla, whipped frosting
1 tbsp rum extract
1 cup toasted coconut

Preheat the oven to 350. Place your coconut (toast the whole bag) on a baking sheet for about 5-7 minutes. Be careful: it browns quickly. Remove from the oven and set to the side. Lightly flour or spray your 9", round cake pans. In a bowl, combine your cake mix, water, rum, oil, toasted coconut, and pineapple juice. Blend on low for about 1 minute, and then on medium for 2 minutes. Pour the batter into the 2 cake pans and place in the oven for 25-30 minutes. Once it is done, remove and let it cool for about 1 hour. In a small sauce pan, bring to a boil your syrup (1/2 cup pineapple juice and 1/2 cup sugar). Using a long-tined fork (or the other end of a wooden spoon) poke large holes all over the cake. Pour the syrup over the cake so it gets moist and infused with flavor. Let it sit in the refrigerator for about 2 hours until you frost it. Once cooled, take your icing and add the rum, stirring it together. Remove cakes from pan and place on a cake dish. Ice your bottom cake very thinly. Then take your pineapple cake fill and put a small layer on top of the cake. Place your other cake on top and frost it as well. At this point, frost the entire cake.

Top with the rest of the toasted coconut and refrigerate for another hour. Decorate as you wish and serve.

FIT CUISINE NOTES:

My mother and I made this dessert for a charity bake off. We wanted to do something fun and different, combining our favorite flavors. We won second place, and it was the most requested recipe of the 12 bakers. Although stressful to make at first, it was really easy and filled with moist flavor.

Time: 2 hours 45 minutes
Serving: 10-12 small pieces

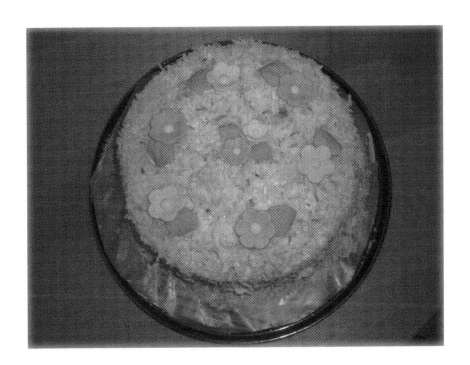

Coconut Cake

Coconut Cookies

WHAT YOU WILL NEED:

1 (14 oz) bag shaved coconut (about 4 cups)
1 medium size can sweetened condensed milk
1 tbsp mini semi-sweet chocolate chips

Preheat the oven to 400. In a large bowl, combine the coconut and the entire can of condensed milk. Using your hands, mix the coconut and milk together, making sure all the coconut is covered. Toss 1/2 tsp of chips in and mix. Using parchment, place your cookies on a baking dish—about 1" apart. Measure the size of your cookies by using a tbsp—each cookie should be the size of one tbsp (you may have to use your hands to fix them). Before you place your cookies in the oven, throw some chips on top. Bake for about 15 minutes (or until the tops are slightly brown). Remove and chill in the refrigerator for 30 minutes.

FIT CUISINE NOTES:

I love coconut, and it's becoming a new healthy food—as long as you don't pair it with heavy creams and butter. I came up with this cookie after sharing coconut cream pie with my husband at our favorite restaurant. This is a portioned, low-calorie way to feel like you are eating a coconut pie. The only difference is, this recipe calls for a little bit of chocolate. I think this is a great, simple, clean cookie that can be made for the family or guests.

Time: 30 minutes
Serving: 16-20 cookies

Applesauce

WHAT YOU WILL NEED:

5-8 apples (any variety you like), sliced
1 tbsp cinnamon

Take all your apples and slice them (keeping the skin on because it contains all the nutrients). Place them in a pot of water and let the water come to a boil (until apples are soft). It should be about 10 minutes. Drain your apples and put them back into your pot. Using a masher, blender, or food processor, spoon your apples into the processor, sprinkle in your cinnamon, and pulse until everything is smooth. Once you are done, place into a container and refrigerate for 1 hour.

FIT CUISINE NOTES:

I love applesauce. I ate it all the time as a kid. Now it seems that all the sauces sold in stores are filled with added sugar and preservatives. So I made this applesauce knowing everything I was eating was natural and healthy. It goes really well with oatmeal or as a midday snack. The kids will love this dish.

Time: 30 minutes
Serving: 6-10

Baked Apple Crisp

WHAT YOU WILL NEED:

4-5 apples sliced (I used Gala)
1 tbsp organic, raw brown sugar
1-2 packets instant cinnamon roll oatmeal
1 tsp dried cranberries
Cooking spray

Preheat the oven to 375. Take a baking dish and spray it. Place your sliced apples on the dish and layer them all around, sprinkling your sugar, oatmeal packet, and cranberries on top. Place in the oven for 15 minutes and serve.

FIT CUISINE NOTES:

This is what I like to call a last-minute, pantry-dessert surprise. It came out really well. I added the leftovers crunch to my yogurt parfait. The flavors of the oatmeal, brown sugar, and apples taste great together. If you are making this dessert, get some low-fat frozen yogurt or ice cream to go with it.

Time: 25 minutes
Serving: 4-6

Dark Chocolate Chip Cookies

WHAT YOU WILL NEED:

3/4 cup rolled oats
1 cup whole wheat flour
1/4 cup I Can't Believe It's Not Butter
1 egg
1/3 cup organic cane sugar
1/3 cup organic brown sugar
1/4 cup canola oil
1/2 tsp baking soda
1 cup dark chocolate chips
1 tsp vanilla extract

Preheat oven to 375. Take your oats and chop them up in a processor (be careful: I have spilled mine all over the counter before). In a small bowl, combine your processed oats, wheat flour, and baking soda and mix together. Then add your sugars, egg, vanilla, oil, and soft butter. Mix together until everything is completely combined. Add chips for the final stir. Line a baking sheet with parchment paper and place your cookie dough on the sheet. Bake for about 20 minutes and let cool.

FIT CUISINE NOTES: 🖊

I am a cookie nut, and I think it makes the perfect dessert—especially if you measure your dough out with a cookie scoop. All you need is one to enjoy the sweet flavors that this cookie has to offer. I wanted to add a twist to the traditional chocolate chip cookie, so I used dark chocolate instead of semi-sweet (for the extra antioxidant benefits). This was easy and yummy and totally worth making again for the kids, a party or to enjoy yourself.

Time: 30 minutes
Serving: 12-18

Bunny Cupcakes

WHAT YOU WILL NEED:

2 cupcake cake mixes
1 container white frosting
1 bag coconut
1 bag large marshmallows
1 small bag jelly beans
1 small bag Peanut M&M's
1 pink gel icing
1 black gel icing
1 container pink sprinkles
Toothpicks or lollipop sticks

Cook your cupcakes according to package. Let them cool before decorating. Set up 1 bowl for your coconut, 1 for your sprinkles, 1 for your M&M's, and 1 for your jelly beans. This way, it is easy to get to the ingredients. Take a knife and slice your marshmallow in half. Stick your toothpick or lollipop stick inside so it is easy to place on the cake.

1. Frost your cooled cupcake
2. Dip in coconut
3. Take your marshmallow ears and dip them in pink sprinkles before placing them on the cupcake
4. Take jelly beans and apply eyes
5. Take M&M's and make a nose
6. Use your black gel icing to make eyes and a mouth
7. Use your pink gel icing to make whiskers

FIT CUISINE NOTES: ✎

My family has certain traditions during the holidays and, for Easter, the Bunny Cake always makes an appearance. I was assigned the job of making this cake each year, but one year I wanted to do a variation on this family tradition. I decided to make the bunny cake have babies. This way, everyone could have a taste without feeling so guilty about eating a large piece of cake. I used all the same flavors and textures; just in a smaller size. It was a family hit, and the babies are here to stay. It is a great dish to make with the family—everyone can design their own bunny.

Time: 1 1/2 hours
Serving: 24 bunnies

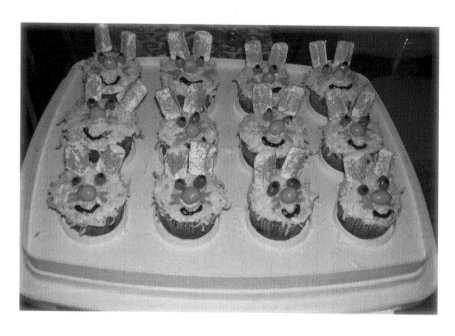

Bunny Cupcakes

Fresh Fruit with Yogurt Dressing and Angel Food Cake

WHAT YOU WILL NEED:

1 cup fat-free Greek yogurt
1 tsp honey
1/2 tsp cinnamon
1 banana, sliced in circles
4 strawberries, sliced in half
2 tbsps raspberries
2 tbsps blueberries
1 store-bought angel food cake, sliced

In a small bowl, combine your yogurt, honey, and cinnamon—making sure all ingredients are stirred together well. Place your angel food cake on a dish and put your fruit on top. Drizzle with the yogurt sauce and serve.

FIT CUISINE NOTES:

This is a light, refreshing dessert that takes no time to prepare. Since I am not a fancy baker, I used store-bought cake (or you can use the box mix). What is great about angel food is the fact that it's fat-free, really airy, and very satisfying (even with just a small piece). It's especially great this way: paired with fruit and yogurt. I taught clients how to make this dish at a party, and it was a hit.

Time: 30-35 minutes
Serving: 6-8

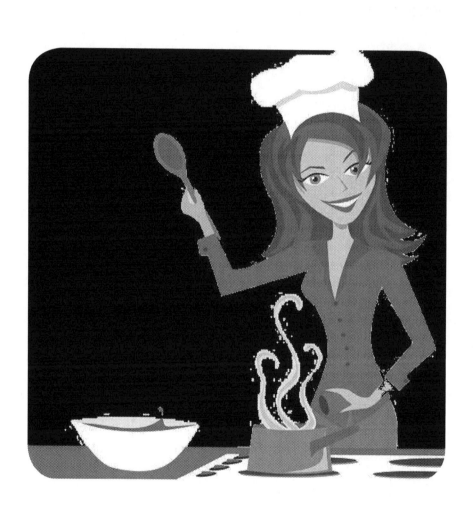

Fit Cuisine Grocery Items

Below are items you should keep on hand to prepare your weekly meals.

- Instant Oatmeal (no sugar like Quaker Plain)
- Kashi (Heart to Heart Cereal Honey Toasted or Sunshine Puffs)

Vegetables and Salad:
ALL KINDS FRESH OR FROZEN

- Anise
- Asparagus
- Zucchini
- Squash
- Green Beans
- Broccoli
- Spinach
- Mushrooms

Fruit:
ALL KINDS FRESH OR FROZEN

Dairy Products/Substitute:

- Milk (non-fat, 1%; skim)
- Almond Milk (unsweetened)
- Goat Cheese (crumbles)
- Low Moisture Mozzarella (shredded)
- Grated Parmesan Cheese
- Cottage Cheese (low salt, low fat)
- Chobani or Fage Greek Yogurt (0%)
- Low Fat Ricotta Cheese
- Feta Cheese (crumbles)
- Blue Cheese (crumbles)

Eggs:

- Regular Eggs
- Liquid Egg substitute
- Liquid Egg Whites

Bread/Pasta/Grains:

- Brown Rice (microwavable found in the freezer isles as well)
- Whole Grain Pasta (Barilla Pasta Plus or Whole Grain)
- Quinoa
- Bulgur
- Couscous
- Tortilla (small)
- Whole Grain Crackers

Meat/Meat Substitute:

- Chicken (breast, thigh, tenders or ground)
- Turkey (breast, ground, tenderloin, cutlets)
- Canned Turkey or Chicken (water packed)
- Tofu (extra firm, or firm)
- Whole Roasted Chicken

Seafood:

- Salmon
- Tuna
- Shrimp
- Scallops
- Mahi Mahi
- Halibut

Nuts:

- Walnuts
- Pine Nuts
- Almonds

- Pistachios
- Dates
- Pecans

Legumes:
ALL Varieties

Canned Items:

- Sliced Beets
- Olives
- Diced Tomatoes (low salt; basil garlic or fire roasted)
- Petite Diced Tomato
- Artichokes (water, olive oil)
- Mandarin Oranges
- Low Fat/Low Sodium Vegetable or Chicken Broth
- Low Sodium Soups (Progresso, Amy's, Healthy Valley)

Extra Staples:

- Tubed Pesto
- Marinara Sauce
- Sliced Sun-dried Tomato
- Fresh Salsa (pineapple/or peach)
- Lemon Juice
- Light Salad Dressing (Italian or Balsamic)
- All Natural Peanut Butter (Skippy, Jiff)
- All Natural Fruit Spread
- Corn Flake crumbles
- Jarred Roasted Red Pepper

Spices and Oils:

- Garlic Powder
- Cumin
- Ms. Dash Tomato Basil Garlic
- Ms. Dash Italian Medley
- Ms. Dash Lemon Pepper

- Ms. Dash Lime Cilantro
- Ginger
- Turmeric
- Cinnamon
- Coriander
- Mint
- Black Pepper
- Red Pepper Flakes
- Basil
- Thyme
- Curry
- Olive Oil
- Balsamic Vinegar
- Cooking Sprays
- Canola Oil
- Vegetable Oil
- Red Wine Vinegar
- Rice Vinegar